The Traumatized Brain

The
Traumatized
BRAIN

A Family Guide to Understanding Mood, Memory, and Behavior after Brain Injury

VANI RAO, MBBS, MD, and
SANDEEP VAISHNAVI, MD, PhD

Foreword by Peter V. Rabins, MD, MPH

Johns Hopkins University Press

Baltimore

This book was brought to publication with the generous assistance of the J. G. Goellner Endowment.

Note to the Reader: This book is not meant to substitute for medical care of people with traumatic brain injury, and treatment should not be based solely on its contents. Instead, treatment must be developed in a dialogue between the individual and his or her physician. Our book has been written to help with that dialogue.

Drug dosage: The author and publisher have made reasonable efforts to determine that the selection of drugs discussed in this text conforms to the practices of the general medical community. The medications described do not necessarily have specific approval by the U.S. Food and Drug Administration for use in the diseases for which they are recommended. In view of ongoing research, changes in governmental regulation, and the constant flow of information relating to drug therapy and drug reactions, the reader is urged to check the package insert of each drug for any change in indications and dosage and for warnings and precautions. This is particularly important when the recommended agent is a new and/or infrequently used drug.

Johns Hopkins University Press
2715 North Charles Street
Baltimore, Maryland 21218-4363
www.press.jhu.edu

Library of Congress Cataloging-in-Publication Data
Rao, Vani, 1958–
    The traumatized brain : a family guide to understanding mood, memory, and behavior after brain injury / by Vani Rao, MBBS, MD, and Sandeep Vaishnavi, MD, PhD ; foreword by Peter V. Rabins, MD, MPH.
        pages cm. — (A Johns Hopkins Press Health Book)
    Includes index.
    ISBN 978-1-4214-1795-0 (pbk. : alk. paper) — ISBN 978-1-4214-1796-7 (electronic) — ISBN 1-4214-1795-2 (pbk. : alk. paper) — ISBN 1-4214-1796-0 (electronic)   1. Brain damage—Complications.   2. Brain damage—Patients—Rehabilitation.   3. Head—Wounds and injuries—Complications.   4. Head—Wounds and injuries—Patients—Rehabilitation.
    I. Vaishnavi, Sandeep, 1973–   II. Rabins, Peter V., writer of foreword.   III. Title.
    RC387.5.R36 2015
    617.4'81044—dc23   2015002495

A catalog record for this book is available from the British Library.

Figures 1.1, 2.1a, 2.1b, 3.1, and 3.2 are by Jacqueline Schaffer.

Special discounts are available for bulk purchases of this book. For more information, please contact Special Sales at 410-516-6936 or specialsales@press.jhu.edu.

Johns Hopkins University Press uses environmentally friendly book materials, including recycled text paper that is composed of at least 30 percent post-consumer waste, whenever possible.

To our patients with brain injury, who continuously educate and motivate us to do better

CONTENTS

Foreword, by Peter V. Rabins   ix
Acknowledgments   xi

Introduction 1

Part I Brain Structure, Function, and Recovery 7
1 The Inner Workings of the Brain 9
2 The Structure of the Brain 15
3 Types of Traumatic Brain Injury 21
4 Influences on Recovery after Traumatic Brain Injury 29

Part II Emotional Problems Caused by the Traumatized Brain 37
5 Depression 39
6 Anxiety 57
7 Mania 66
8 Apathy 72

Part III Behavioral Problems Caused by the Traumatized Brain 79
9 Psychosis 81
10 Aggression 89
11 Impulsivity 99
12 Sleep Disturbances 106

Part IV Cognitive Problems Caused by the Traumatized Brain 117
13 Attention 119
14 Memory 125

15 Executive Function 133

16 Language 140

**Part V Other Common Problems Caused by
the Traumatized Brain 147**

17 Headaches 149

18 Seizures 155

19 Vision 163

Epilogue 171

Glossary   179
Resources   185
Suggested Reading   189
Index   191

Traumatic brain injury (TBI) is not a new health care issue, but improvements in trauma care have led to the survival of many severely injured people who are left with the aftermath of an injured brain. In addition, research and clinical experience show that head injuries that in the past were considered insignificant or minor have adverse long-term outcomes.

These changes have occurred in community hospitals, on the battlefield, and on the playing field, and these injuries have been compounded by the development of new ways of inflicting injury. The Iraq and Afghanistan wars have seen the wide use of improvised explosive devices (IEDs) that appear to cause injury through the generation of a large pressure wave, which leads to "internal" damage in people near a blast. These brain injuries have often occurred in addition to the penetrating wounds that have long been the consequence of war. In the civilian world, the development of "protective" helmets, seat belts, and improved trauma care have led to more survivors with TBI but also more mood, cognitive, and behavior consequences.

The renewed focus on TBI has led to the realization that we know relatively little about the mechanisms of such injuries and even less about how best to treat people who have experienced them. The recognition that TBI is much more widespread and disabling than was appreciated in the past has been paralleled by the realization that those with TBI require specialized care by knowledgeable professionals. Although it is unfortunate that it has taken a set of tragedies to bring attention to the long-smoldering problem of TBI, the realization of its serious public health impact has resulted in gains in knowledge and long overdue support for clinical care.

In *The Traumatized Brain: A Family Guide to Understanding Mood, Memory, and Behavior after Brain Injury*, Vani Rao and Sandeep Vaishnavi bring to the care of people with TBI an intimate knowledge of the function of the healthy brain, a knowledge of the types of injury associated with TBI, and a critical examination of management of chronic problems associated with TBI. As experienced clinicians who care for people with TBI, Drs. Rao and Vaishnavi are able to bring a practical eye to this merging of advances in research, clinical knowledge, and awareness of the science supporting the efficacy of available nondrug and drug treatments.

This book will challenge and encourage the reader. Whether an interested lay person, a caretaker, a family member, or a professional in the medical, nursing, or social work fields, the reader will find this pioneering book a useful guide to the complexities of TBI.

Peter V. Rabins, MD, MPH
Baltimore, Maryland

ACKNOWLEDGMENTS

The inspiration for this book comes from *The 36-Hour Day*, written by Nancy L. Mace and Peter V. Rabins. I read that book as a resident, and I was blown away by the authors' descriptions of a very complex disease such as Alzheimer's disease in simple segments intended to educate caregivers and give them hope. My heartfelt gratitude goes to Dr. Rabins not only for motivating me but also for the relentless support he gave Sandeep and me as we worked on this book.

I am most grateful to Dr. Constantine Lyketsos, my mentor and guide, for his consistent encouragement from the start of this book to its completion. I am truly indebted to him.

Two dear friends, Dr. Sasikala Vemuri, an internist in Michigan, and Ms. Joelle Ridgeway, health care administrator in the field of brain injury, also provided tremendous help as we worked through the manuscript by meticulously reviewing and commenting on earlier drafts. To them I extend my utmost appreciation.

I am much obliged and thankful to Ms. Jacqueline Wehmueller, Executive Editor, Johns Hopkins University Press, for her support, encouragement, and feedback and for helping us bring this book to fruition. Special thanks go to Ms. Molly Ward and Ms. Barbara Lamb for their skillful review and guidance, and to Ms. Jacqueline Schaffer for turning our simple pencil drawings into beautiful illustrations. This book would not have been completed without the guidance and assistance of this team.

Over the course of years, there have been many teachers, friends, and colleagues who have stood by me and backed me with their support, assistance, and positive comments. I will forever be thankful for their help. I am especially grateful to all who have shaped my career through my interactions with them and their clinical and research work. They include Drs. Gwenn Smith, Vassilis Koliatsos, Kathleen Bechtold, Jason Brandt, Robert Robinson, Ricardo Jorge, Jonathan Silver, David Arciniegas, Thomas McAllister, and Jesse Fann.

It has been a pleasure working with my coauthor, Sandeep, who stimulated me and kept me on my toes as we worked on this book.

To my patients, from whom I have learned most of what I know about the neuropsychiatric consequences of TBI, I shall ever be grateful.

Finally, without my family this book would never have been started. My eternal gratitude goes to my parents, Professor Santappa and Mrs. Dhanalakshmi Devi, my pillars of strength, for raising me to believe in myself, to my husband, Narsima, for being "the wind beneath my wings," to my children, Veena and Harsha Vardhan, for inspiring and cheering me along as I have journeyed through my career, and to my siblings, Shyla, Sunanda, Umesh, and Ravi, and their spouses/children for their constant kind words of support.

Vani Rao

I would like to thank my mentors and teachers at Johns Hopkins, where I did part of my medical training, including my coauthor, Dr. Vani Rao. I will be forever indebted for their guidance. I would also like to acknowledge the patience and guidance of my wife, Deepti, as I worked on this book. My young children, Shivum and Dhruv, have continuously helped remind me of the curiosity about the world we are all born with. I would also like to express my deep gratitude to my grandfather, S. L. (Shyam Lal) Vaishnavi, who first introduced me to the possibility of writing about science for the general public with his book, *The Nature of Reality*. Finally, I wish to acknowledge my parents, Dr. Vijay and Kirti Vaishnavi. Without their infinite patience and support and guidance, I certainly would not have been in a position to write this book.

Sandeep Vaishnavi

We would like to thank Ms. Anastasia Edmonston, Project Director, TBI and Person Centered Planning Trainer, Maryland Mental Hygiene Administration, who helped us compile the resource guide.

Also, in this book, we provide specific suggestions for patients and family members. These are suggestions we make when we talk to our own patients and their family members, but we would like to acknowledge the significant contributions made by other traumatic brain injury clinicians and researchers. This book is the result of all of our collective wisdom, and we appreciate the education and teachings we have had from our mentors and colleagues.

All cases in this book are compositions of patients we have taken care of. Patients' personal histories have been changed and clinical details modified to ensure confidentiality and privacy. We thank them for the opportunity we have had to serve them.

VR, SV

The Traumatized Brain

Introduction

THIS BOOK IS ABOUT BRAIN INJURY. There are many different types of brain injury, but here we focus on injuries caused by trauma (such as a car accident, a fall, a battle injury, or a blow to the head suffered in amateur or professional sports). A brain injury caused by trauma is known as traumatic brain injury, or TBI.

Traumatic brain injuries are classified as mild, moderate, or severe, based on how long the person was unconscious or how much time passed before he or she could make new memories. Most people with mild TBI make a spontaneous recovery within the first few months of injury. But mild brain injuries are not always benign, especially if there have been multiple injuries over the years.

Each type of traumatic brain injury has its own consequences, from acute to chronic, from mild to severe. In this book, we draw on our experiences in treating those with brain injury to explain what happens with these injuries. Of course, each person's experience is different, depending on many factors—the severity of injury, other injuries the person may have suffered, medical problems, medications, use of illicit drugs, the person's personality traits and genetic vulnerability. We address both mild and moderate to severe brain injuries. The common theme is our focus on long-term consequences. Although traditional thinking has been that moderate to severe injuries lead to long-term consequences, there is some emerging evidence that repeated mild injuries may also affect a person in the long term. Such repeated mild injuries may occur in the context of contact sports such as football, especially professional football, but even perhaps with amateur (school and college) football, as well as soccer, boxing, and other contact sports.

Traumatic brain injuries have a huge impact, both literally and figuratively. People with TBI may suffer not only from the immediate consequences of the injury, such as the potential for bleeding in the brain or for seizures, but also from long-term problems, which are often related to changes in mood, thinking, attention, memory, and behavior. These long-term consequences can be confusing to family and friends who may think that their loved one with brain injury has changed but be unable to understand why.

Traumatic brain injuries are in a sense a silent epidemic, because often, after persons with TBI have been treated in the emergency department or released from the hospital, family members or friends may assume that they are now "fixed." There may be no physical evidence of injury, so it is easy for others to believe that everything is back to normal. Unfortunately, that is often not the case, especially with more severe injuries.

We spend much of the book discussing the long-term effects after TBI, particularly the emotional, cognitive, and behavioral symptoms, regardless of the cause, whether a severe brain injury or the result of many repeated mild injuries. We do so because these symptoms are often not well recognized and continue to be distressing to both the person with brain injury and his or her family. These symptoms, often called neuropsychiatric (or more generally, psychiatric) symptoms, are often the symptoms that have the greatest impact on quality of life. If these symptoms are not recognized by the person with the brain injury and his or her family, misunderstandings are sure to follow.

The person with TBI may not be able to function well because of these symptoms, so relationships and employment suffer because the person is unable to achieve his or her full potential. These outcomes are particularly tragic because many of these symptoms are treatable. The brain is traumatized physically by brain injury, but physical trauma can lead to emotional consequences—even emotional trauma. Furthermore, family members themselves may be emotionally traumatized; they may not understand why their loved one has changed so much and may not know how to even begin to help.

Our aim in this book is to give voice to this silent epidemic and everyone affected by it. We want to help readers recognize and understand the psychiatric symptoms that develop after TBI. Unlike physical symptoms, such as a change in appearance or a change in one's ability to get around, psychiatric symptoms are often overlooked or misunderstood. Recognizing the symptoms is the first step in addressing them. Here we discuss in general some of the medication treatments that have proven to be helpful. We also advise the reader on general actions to take and some behavioral methods to use to minimize psychiatric symptoms after TBI. (A *note of caution:* This book should not and cannot be used for self-treatment of traumatic brain injury. The services of a medical professional are essential for appropriate treatment.)

Finally, we hope to explain why psychiatric symptoms are real and how they can result from damage to certain parts of the brain, as happens in TBI. Unfortunately, a stigma still surrounds psychiatric symptoms, stemming from the mistaken belief that they are not as "real" as physical symptoms. But psychiatric symptoms in TBI are as real as physical symptoms—indeed, they are symptoms of damage to higher-order areas of the brain, to specific brain circuits. Just as people with sensory problems (like blindness) or motor deficits (like paralysis) have damage to certain circuits that neurologists focus on, people with psychiatric symptoms have damage to other circuits, to those that modulate our mood, control our impulses, manage our memories, and allow us to act in a socially appropriate manner and to think.

This book is divided into five parts. In the first part, we discuss how the brain works. To explain brain injury, we provide an overview describing the structure and functioning of the normal brain as well as the impact of trauma. We feel it is important to present in some detail how damage to the brain can lead to psychiatric symptoms, both to get a better theoretical understanding of how psychiatric and physical symptoms are equally real and to get a better practical understanding of brain injury. Given the nature of the topic, these chapters are somewhat technical. You can skip the first part of the book if you wish to focus on symptoms and how best to manage them. If you are inclined, though, reading through the first section may be rewarding, giving you a richer idea of what happens with brain injury.

We devote much of the rest of the chapters to explaining the major emotional, behavioral, and cognitive issues that can arise after TBI. In these chapters, we present typical case examples (which, to protect privacy, are composites of actual cases) and discuss in greater detail how damage to particular areas of the brain can lead to the symptoms you may see in your loved one. When we discuss how brain damage in certain areas leads to certain symptoms, we are simplifying the science. Our descriptions of the brain structures and circuitry are first approximations only, reflecting current ways to think about what is going on in the brain. We are by no means giving a definitive account of brain pathophysiology, but we have tried to provide a framework or model, even if it is an approximation and primitive, of how to connect brain structure and function with brain injury and dysfunction.

We include specific medication and nonmedication treatments to help patients and their families. Wherever medications are mentioned, we provide the brand name, followed by the generic name in parentheses: for example, Zoloft (sertraline). We conclude each chapter with a summary of specific behavioral methods you can use to help manage symptoms in brain injury.

Research in science and medicine is going on all the time, and in the future, we will know more about how the brain does what it does, and we will be able to help those who suffer from brain injuries even more than we can today. But we already understand a great deal. We understand that psychiatric symptoms are part of brain injury, we accept that psychiatric symptoms after brain injury cause significant problems, and we know that these symptoms can

> *Note*: No person should take a prescription medication unless a licensed physician has specifically prescribed it for him or her after proper medical evaluation. No person should take a medication, adjust the dose of a medication, or stop taking a medication without first consulting his or her physician. Any person taking a prescription medication should be supervised and monitored by a physician for the duration of the prescription.

indeed be managed. The more we know, the more hope there is for patients and their families and friends. Many people with TBI are suffering in silence because they are misunderstood. We hope this book sheds light on their condition and brings help to persons with brain injury and their families as they embark on a journey of recovery of the traumatized brain.

Both males and females, of course, suffer traumatic brain injury. In Chapters 4 through 19 of this book, we use male or female patients in the chapter-opening stories and corresponding masculine or feminine pronouns in the text.

PART I

Brain Structure, Function, and Recovery

In this section of the book, we focus on brain structure and function. We do so for a few reasons, but primarily because it can
be useful to understand how the brain operates so that the effects
of damage to the brain make more sense. After all, to understand
dysfunction, it is helpful to understand normal function. We try to
minimize extraneous detail and excessive technicality, but you can
certainly skip this section if you wish. You may want to use this
section as a reference to come back to as needed.

In Chapter 1, we look at the brain at a cellular level. We introduce a number of words necessary to communicate about the
brain. This may be helpful to readers who wish to understand the
medical terminology used by doctors (see also "Glossary").
In Chapter 2, we look at the brain at a structural level, that is, at
different parts of the brain. We focus in this chapter, as we do
throughout, on parts of the brain that are involved with mood,
behavior, and cognitive processing. In Chapter 3, we build on the
first two chapters and make the transition from normal function
to dysfunction, from normality to pathology. We discuss different
types of brain injury and their impact on different aspects of the

brain. Finally, in Chapter 4, we discuss how the brain can recover; we explain that the brain is always dynamic, always learning, always malleable—characteristics that are the basis of the behavioral advice we give in parts of the book where we discuss how to improve specific symptoms after brain injury.

1

The Inner Workings of the Brain

THE BRAIN IS A REMARKABLE ORGAN—a three-pound mass of ge-latinous material that allows us to be who we are. It allows us to re-member, speak, think, plan, and move. It allows us to have our unique personalities, our emotions, and our dreams for the future.

At a fundamental level, the brain houses our sense of self, of who we are. If you were to ask people to point to the part of the body that makes them who they are, would they point to their liver, their lungs, or their kidneys? Most likely not. Most people would point to their brains.

We have an intuitive sense that the brain is unique among all the organs of the body. It does indeed have a privileged position: it is in many ways the conductor, the maestro, coordinating the orches-tra of the body. Through its connections to the nerves and the spinal cord, the brain controls the beating of our heart, the digestion in our gastrointestinal tract, the workings of our lungs. Even more funda-mentally, the brain allows us to be awake, conscious, and aware.

Despite its unique position, the brain is part of a larger system, the nervous system. The nervous system itself consists of distinct systems: the central nervous system and the peripheral nervous system, which includes the autonomic nervous system. The central nervous system is composed of the brain and the spinal cord. The peripheral nervous system includes the nerve roots that come out of the spinal cord (known as spinal roots), the peripheral nerves, and a region where nerves meet muscles, called the neuromuscular junction. The autonomic nervous system is itself subdivided into sympathetic and parasympathetic components, which control functions we don't have to think about, including our heartbeat, breathing, and digestion. Another way to think about the nervous system is to divide it into components that, when damaged, lead to specific signs and symptoms of malfunction or disease. In this way of thinking, we can separate the nervous system into units: the cerebral cortex, the cerebellum, the brainstem, the spinal cord, the spinal roots, the peripheral nerves, and the neuromuscular junction. The cerebral cortex, the cerebellum, and the brainstem are in the brain itself.

The brain's fundamental unit of operation is the brain cell, called a neuron (figure 1.1). There are a lot of neurons in the human brain, something on the order of 100 billion. In addition to neurons, the brain features other cells, called glial cells. We used to think that glial cells were only there to support neurons, but it may be that glial cells do more than that—they may also, like neurons, contribute to the brain's computing power (and may even outnumber neurons).

The body of a neuron is called the soma. Attached to the soma are branches called dendrites and axons. Dendrites receive signals from other neurons. Axons are long sheaths that lead up to the space between neurons. The space between any two given neurons is called the synapse.

Neurons are electrochemical units, meaning that they depend on both electric current and chemicals to function. The chemical process depends on the concentration of particles of sodium, potassium, chloride, and calcium. Differing concentrations of these particles inside and outside the neuron create voltage differences across the neuron membrane (the outer "skin" of the cell). When sodium or potassium enters the neuron, these voltage differences become less negatively charged. When this difference becomes less negative enough, the neuron fires, meaning that electrical current flows across the neuron and down an axon. When the electrical current reaches

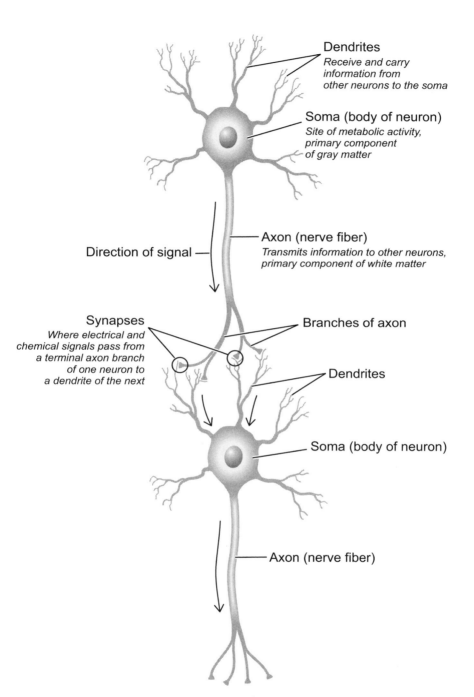

Figure 1.1. Normal neurons

the end of the axon, a group of chemicals called neurotransmitters flow into the synapse. These neurotransmitters include the chemicals serotonin, norepinephrine, dopamine, glutamate, and gamma-aminobutyric acid (GABA). Once the neurotransmitters are released, they lock onto receptors on the next neuron. This coupling then changes the voltage of that neuron, making it, in turn, more or less likely to fire. This is a simplistic explanation of what happens in the brain. In reality, each neuron has input from multiple other neurons at its dendrites, perhaps at the same time. Whether a certain neuron fires or not, whether it excites or inhibits the next neuron, is based on complex dynamics.

Neurons group together into pathways, or circuits, that carry out certain functions. For example, one circuit, called the corticospinal tract, allows us to move our body. The corticospinal tract begins in the motor cortex in the brain, travels through the brainstem into the spinal cord, and then through peripheral nerves to the muscles. This circuit thus includes a large number of neurons, all communicating and coordinating with one another by means of electricity and chemicals. The corticospinal tract is categorized as a motor circuit.

Sensory circuits allow us to sense information in the environment. There are separate circuits for pain, temperature, touch, vibration, vision, hearing, smell, taste, and more. Coordination circuits control how we coordinate our movements, allowing us to move fluidly.

In addition to the motor, sensory, and coordination circuits, the brain has a number of more complex circuits that can be called higher-order circuits. These circuits regulate our mood, thinking, memory, impulse control, and personality, among other things. They control what we think of as "selves," the qualities that make us human, that make us who we are. Underlying this are circuits that control consciousness itself, the ability to be awake and conscious.

The idea that these higher-order circuits are responsible for creating who we are is a fundamental but controversial concept. We may hesitate at some level to believe that there are circuits in the brain that make up our personality, our motivations, our intentions—

the qualities that make "us" us. Most people have no difficulty believing that there are circuits that control movements or sense the environment, but they may hesitate to think that the qualities that make us who we are, make us individuals, are also housed in brain circuitry. A fundamental tenet of modern neuroscience (the scientific study of the nervous system) is that damage to these higher-order circuits results in psychiatric symptoms such as depression, anxiety, memory loss, and abnormal behavior. Traumatic brain injury can damage these very circuits, affecting those who suffer from TBI in fundamental ways.

We like to believe that we are more than our circuits and that we have a sense of control over our destinies. We all believe that we have intention and can come up with a plan and then execute that plan. Perhaps we can. However, to do all of this, the infrastructure of the brain, particularly that higher-order circuitry, must be intact. Without that intact infrastructure, our intentions and plans cannot be carried out the way we want them to. A common analogy is with computer hardware and software. We may have the most sophisticated software program, but if we are running it on a damaged computer, we cannot take advantage of the software. Similarly, if the hardware of the brain is not intact, we cannot have our emotions, our plans, our dreams.

Clearly then, to understand the software of our behavior, we have to understand the hardware that is the brain. By focusing on the brain and its circuitry, we are not minimizing the human condition. Humans are not automatons, passively dependent on chemicals in the brain. Our view in this book is that there is no contradiction between our sense that we are more than our brains and the neuroscientific view that our perceptions of ourselves and the world are based on brain circuitry. We do agree that our thinking, emotions, and behavior are dependent on both nature and nurture; the development of our brain circuitry is based on genes and the environment we interact with.

Our brain is changing all the time, as we interact with our environment, as we react to new information. Our brain has to be dynamic or we would not do very well in a constantly changing world.

Humans have evolved to a point where we dominate other species largely because our brains are so dynamic and adaptable. This dynamism is also reflected in our brain circuitry.

So, all the richness and complexity of our mental lives, our moods, our behaviors, our thinking and memory, are based on the interaction of brain circuits laid down as our brains developed as babies and on changes to these circuits as we accumulated environmental experiences. In other words, we are not who we are only because our brains were fated to develop in a certain way, and we are not who we are only because of the environments in which we find ourselves. We are who we are because of a combination of both—of nature and nurture.

This notion is similar to current thinking about our genetic code. Our DNA does not doom us inevitably to develop certain illnesses. Of course, our genetic code does predispose us to particular illnesses because it reflects contributions from our genetic predecessors. However, environmental factors, both good and bad, can affect how these genes are expressed. By changing our behavior—exercising, eating certain foods, and perhaps taking certain medications—we may be able to change how our genes are expressed. There is even emerging evidence that the bacteria and viruses we carry in our bodies (called the microbiome) can affect how our genes are expressed.

We can, in some ways, then, change our fate, at least to some degree. Nevertheless, we should be aware of the genetic sequences we are born with because they are the basis of what may happen to us in the future. Similarly, we should understand our brain circuits, because they are the basis of how we are who we are.

In the next chapter, we look at the brain's structures in greater detail. We explore different parts and structures of the brain and discuss what they do. You may skip the next chapter if you feel that the information there is too technical or not relevant at the moment; you can always return to it later. We do hope, though, that you will join us as we explore the structures of the brain, which, in many ways, make us who we are and let us think, feel, dream, remember, and plan.

2

The Structure of the Brain

IN THE LAST CHAPTER we introduced a number of terms and focused on the brain at a cellular and neuronal level. In this chapter, we explore the structure of the brain—the parts of the brain and how they work together. We discuss the major components of the brain, including the cerebral cortex, the cerebellum, the basal ganglia, the thalamus, the hypothalamus, and the brainstem.

The brain consists of two types of tissue: white matter and gray matter. White matter consists of long strands of axons, called axon tracts, which connect the different parts of the brain. White matter carries the signals or messages to different parts of the brain. A layer of fatty tissue called myelin, which protects the axons and helps in signal transmission, covers the axons. The fat in myelin appears white, hence the name white matter.

Gray matter contains the neurons, as well as other supporting cells, including glial cells. Within the gray matter, neurons connect and form synapses. Gray matter contains only cells and small blood vessels and lacks the white myelin.

Although the various regions of the brain connect and work together, structurally the brain is divided into distinct areas, each of

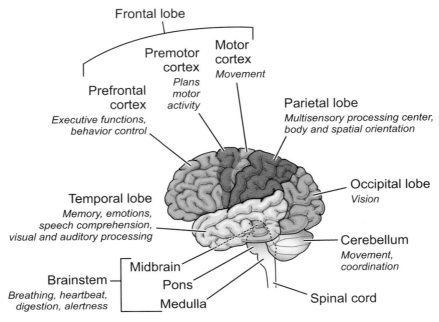

Figure 2.1a. Side view of the brain

which has its unique function. Figures 2.1a and b illustrate the major regions of the brain.

The brainstem is in the back of the brain and connects the brain with the spinal cord. The brainstem is composed of the midbrain, pons, and medulla. The brainstem is critical to life. Groups of cells distributed throughout the brainstem compose a network called the reticular activating system (RAS). The RAS allows us to be conscious, alert, and aware. Damage to the RAS results in unconsciousness.

The lowest section of the brainstem, the medulla, controls critical moment-to-moment automatic functions like breathing and heartbeat. The pons portion of the brainstem plays a role in generating dreams during sleep. Axon tracts carrying sensory and motor information travel through the brainstem to and from the spinal cord, so damage to the brainstem can lead to paralysis or a disturbing condition called locked-in syndrome, in which the person is conscious and aware but is unable to move any portion of the body

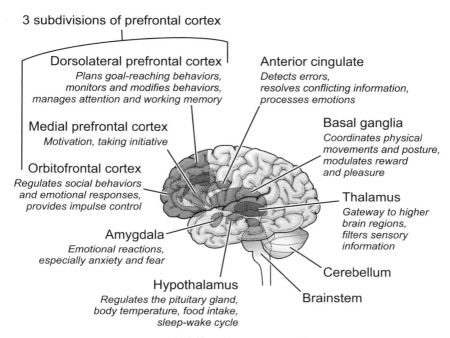

3 subdivisions of prefrontal cortex

Dorsolateral prefrontal cortex
*Plans goal-reaching behaviors,
monitors and modifies behaviors,
manages attention and working memory*

Anterior cingulate
*Detects errors,
resolves conflicting information,
processes emotions*

Medial prefrontal cortex
Motivation, taking initiative

Basal ganglia
*Coordinates physical
movements and posture,
modulates reward
and pleasure*

Orbitofrontal cortex
*Regulates social behaviors
and emotional responses,
provides impulse control*

Thalamus
*Gateway to higher
brain regions,
filters sensory
information*

Amygdala
*Emotional reactions,
especially anxiety and fear*

Cerebellum

Hypothalamus
*Regulates the pituitary gland,
body temperature, food intake,
sleep-wake cycle*

Brainstem

Figure 2.1b. Medial (deep inside) view of the brain

except for the eyes. Because cognitive activities like thinking and memory are not housed in the brainstem, damage to the brainstem does not affect these higher-order functions.

Sitting above the brainstem is the thalamus. The thalamus, in its role as the relay system of sensory information, is a critical part of the brain's interconnected architecture. It receives input from the environment (through vision, hearing, touch), processes it, and then sends it to the rest of the brain. The thalamus filters out "unnecessary" sensory stimuli so that the rest of the brain is not overwhelmed with information. It is involved in thought, which means that people who have damage to the thalamus can be confused and disoriented. The thalamus is also involved in our ability to pay attention, and it plays a role in spatial attention.

Below the thalamus lies the hypothalamus. This portion of the brain is involved in expressing rage and in feeding and sexual behaviors. The hypothalamus controls the nearby pituitary gland, the so-called master gland of the body. The pituitary gland secretes chemicals called hormones, such as growth hormone and thyroid-stimulating hormone, which affect the actions of many body organs.

The cerebellum, at the back of the brain near the brainstem, helps with movement, particularly the ability to coordinate balance. People who have damage to the cerebellum have trouble walking in a straight line. Alcohol can impair the cerebellum, which is why police sobriety tests include walking heel-to-toe and touching the finger to the nose in a smooth, direct fashion. Yet the cerebellum's role is not limited to movement; it may also be involved with the coordination and fluidity of both thought and speech.

Deep within the brain, near the center and bordering the thalamus, lie two sets of structures, called basal ganglia, which are also involved with movement. The basal ganglia are composed of four distinct groups of cells, called nuclei. The four nuclei are the putamen, the caudate, the subthalamic nucleus, and the globus pallidus. Within each set of basal ganglia on either side of the brain, these nuclei form circuits that smoothen out our movements. Parkinson's disease and other movement disorders affect this area of the brain. Damage to the basal ganglia can result in tremor and walking difficulties. The basal ganglia also have important roles in cognition, and several circuits connect the basal ganglia to the frontal lobes of the brain. Part of the basal ganglia (the ventral striatum and, more specifically, the nucleus accumbens) is important for our sense of pleasure and reward.

The cerebral cortex is the outer covering of the brain and consists of many folds and ridges. The cortex is highly developed in humans, and this sophistication is believed to be one critical factor that differentiates humans from other animals. The cortex is composed of four divisions called lobes—the frontal lobe, temporal lobe, parietal lobe, and occipital lobe. There is a duplicate set of lobes on each side of the brain.

The frontal lobe plays an important part in higher-order cognitive activities like thinking, planning, goal-setting, organizing thoughts, abstracting, and conceptualizing. It also is important in organizing movements. The frontal lobe is often known as the chief executive officer of the brain. The frontal lobe consists of the motor cortex, the premotor cortex, and the prefrontal cortex. As their names suggest, the motor cortex and premotor cortex are associated with movement.

The prefrontal cortex itself has three regions: the ventral prefrontal cortex (with the orbitofrontal cortex as the main component), the dorsolateral prefrontal cortex, and the medial prefrontal cortex. The prefrontal cortex is involved in cognitive activity. Damage to the orbitofrontal cortex, which can occur with traumatic brain injury, can lead to significant personality changes; for example, not caring for social conventions and becoming self-centered. Excessive activity in the orbitofrontal cortex can cause repetitive thoughts and behaviors, as happens in obsessive-compulsive disorder. The dorsolateral prefrontal cortex is mainly associated with cognitive functioning, specifically executive functions such as planning, organizing, abstract reasoning, and inhibition, and it contributes to cognitive flexibility and working memory. In addition, in its connections with other regions of the brain, the dorsolateral prefrontal cortex also contributes to mood changes such as depression. The dorsolateral prefrontal cortex is frequently damaged in TBI, creating problems with cognitive activity and mood changes.

The temporal lobes house circuits involved in processing visual and auditory information. Damage to the temporal lobes can lead to visual problems, trouble with hearing, and even auditory hallucinations (as in schizophrenia). In the inside (or medial) part of the temporal lobe, one circuit is involved in short-term memory storage. The medial temporal lobe contains the hippocampus, a crucial structure in memory formation. Alzheimer's disease is associated with damage to the hippocampus. Similarly, people with TBI who have damage to the temporal lobe can have memory problems.

Deeper inside the brain, near the temporal lobe, is a circuit called the limbic system, which regulates our emotions. The limbic system includes the amygdala, the mamillary body, and the anterior cingulate. Research indicates that excess activity in the amygdala is related to high levels of anxiety.

The anterior cingulate seems to be crucial for cognitive functions (for example, detecting errors and resolving conflicts), motivation, and emotional stability. This region may also have a role in the development of anxiety and depressive symptoms. Research suggests that deep-brain stimulation of a special region of the anterior cingulate may be helpful in treating depressive symptoms.

The occipital lobes are important for vision, and damage to them can lead to blindness. Different parts of each of the occipital lobes allow us to recognize shape, visual movement, and color. Visual information, once processed in the occipital lobes, is sent on to the temporal lobes for further analysis; the temporal lobe areas that connect to the occipital lobes help us identify faces and integrate the various attributes of a given object (movement with shape, for example).

In this chapter, we have provided a brief overview of the major parts of the brain. The interconnectedness of the brain makes its function highly complex. Damage to any one area of the brain can set off a string of repercussions to physical, emotional, and cognitive health. We focus on the areas of the brain that are most commonly affected by TBI in Chapter 3, and we discuss different types of brain injury in Chapter 4.

3

Types of Traumatic Brain Injury

TRAUMATIC BRAIN INJURY (TBI) can damage different parts of the brain in many and various ways. Depending on the severity of injury, the consequences of traumatic brain damage range from the absence of symptoms to mild symptoms and sometimes even to death. The severity of symptoms is usually proportional to the severity and type of brain injury. In this chapter, we describe the most common causes of brain injury and how those injuries affect brain tissue. Although the medical words and phrases we introduce here might be overwhelming, we think it is important to be familiar with them because you may have heard them from your doctors. Our aim is to help you understand the bewildering terminology of TBI and give you a better sense of how TBIs can happen.

Types of TBI

The major forms of traumatic brain injury are impact injury, penetrating injury, injury from inertial forces, and blast injury.

An impact injury occurs when the head makes sudden, forceful contact with some object. In an impact injury, the brain accelerates, and then abruptly stops. An example of this is a fall: when a person falls, the brain accelerates as gravity pulls the body down, then suddenly stops when the head hits the ground.

In a penetrating injury, an object penetrates the brain. An example is a bullet that passes through the skull into the brain. The trajectory (path) and speed of the bullet directly damage the brain. Changes in air pressure caused by the traveling bullet can also damage brain tissue. Because they cause direct damage to the brain matter, penetrating injuries can lead to tissue death and irritation of the brain, which can cause seizures.

Injury from inertial forces results when the brain moves within the skull, but not as a result of head impact. An example of this is a car accident in which the head jerks suddenly when the car is hit by another vehicle.

Finally, there is blast injury, which most frequently occurs in the context of war or a bomb explosion. Shock waves from the explosion are believed to be the cause of brain damage because of the sudden change in pressure brought on by the exploding device.

Types of Brain Damage from TBI

Each form of TBI causes distinct types of damage. Similarly, each type of damage has its own unique consequences. Brain tissue can be bruised or torn. Blood can collect between the skull and the brain or within the brain itself. Areas of the brain can be damaged if the brain swells, putting pressure on distinct regions as it tries to expand within the limited confines of the skull. Swelling brain tissue can stretch or press on the delicate nerve fibers that carry messages throughout the body, or it can compress blood vessels, cutting off the oxygen supply to that part of the brain.

Bruises, Cuts, and Skull Fractures

Contusions, or bruising of the brain, commonly occur in impact injuries. The force of the impact "throws" the brain into the skull, damaging the soft tissue. For example, the front of the head hitting a solid object can cause a contusion in the frontal lobes. This impact

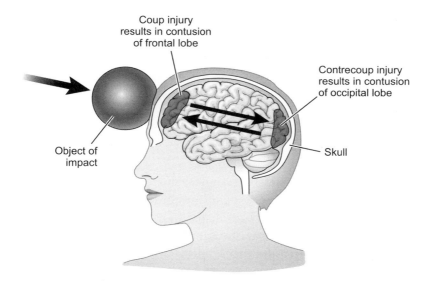

Figure 3.1. Coup-contrecoup injury

is called a coup injury. Coup injuries are often followed immediately by a contrecoup injury, when the impact of the object jostles the brain within the skull, which damages the opposite area of the brain. Figure 3.1 shows a coup-contrecoup injury in the occipital lobe at the back of the brain.

Among the contributors to contusions after a direct hit to the brain are bony areas and ridges on the interior of the skull overlying the frontal and temporal lobes. These irregular surfaces protrude into the skull cavity, making the frontal and temporal lobes more vulnerable to TBI. As discussed elsewhere in this book, damage to the frontal and temporal lobes can cause significant mood, behavioral, and cognitive changes. Damage to these areas may not be immediately obvious to family and friends because the person with the TBI may be able to move and talk normally, but there can be significant changes in personality, that is, a meaningful change from who the person "was" before the injury.

Skull fractures typically result in severe TBIs for several reasons. A particularly forceful head impact can fracture the skull, so the presence of a skull fracture indicates a significant force associated with the trauma. Skull fractures are more likely than other traumas to cause bleeding within the brain. People who sustain a skull fracture may be more likely to develop seizures. The phrase *brain laceration* describes brain tissue that is physically cut or torn, either by the pushed-in bone fragment from a skull fracture or by a foreign object such as a bullet or bullet fragment from a gunshot wound.

Bleeding in the Brain

The medical term for bleeding within the brain is *intracranial hemorrhage*. There are two types of intracranial hemorrhage: those between the brain and the skull (called epidural hemorrhage, subdural hemorrhage, or subarachnoid hemorrhage, based on their location) and those within the brain itself (called intracerebral hemorrhage). The words *hematoma* and *hemorrhage* are easily confused. *Hemorrhage* means active bleeding, whereas *hematoma* means clotted blood or a collection of blood outside a blood vessel (for example, an artery, a vein, or capillaries) into a tissue space such as brain tissue. Hematomas can be small or large. Symptoms from a hematoma depend on its size and whether it is exerting pressure on nearby tissue.

An epidural hematoma is a collection of blood right below the skull, between the skull and a thin outer covering of the brain called the dura mater. We usually see epidural hematomas in the temporal areas, and their cause is often injury to the side of the head. The majority of epidural hematomas are the result of damage to the meningeal arteries, but a small proportion can also be due to damage to veins. Because the blood in all arteries is under higher pressure than blood in veins, leaking blood can quickly accumulate and injure the brain. Epidural hematomas cause brain damage because the pool of leaking blood can press down on the adjacent brain, indenting and flattening it. The result is lack of oxygen (called anoxic injury) in the tissue that is being compressed. Epidural hematomas are almost always medical emergencies.

A subdural hematoma is also a collection of blood between the brain and the skull, but below the dura mater membrane. Subdural hematomas are closer to the brain than epidural hematomas, but they are still outside the brain. Subdural hematomas tend to arise from tears in veins as opposed to arteries, so they accumulate more slowly than epidural hematomas, because veins are under less pressure than arteries. Subdural hematomas develop most often in elderly people, whose veins are more fragile and have stretched because of underlying brain atrophy (shrinkage). Elderly people and people who abuse alcohol are particularly prone to subdural hematomas because they are likely to fall or bump their head. The blood in a subdural hematoma can collect slowly, so the person with this type of injury may not be immediately aware of the injury. Both elderly people and people with chronic alcohol problems may fall repeatedly and suffer repeated subdural hematomas.

A subarachnoid hemorrhage is a collection of blood even closer to the brain than a subdural hematoma, but still outside the brain. Subarachnoid hemorrhages develop below the arachnoid mater— yet another membrane covering the brain—but beneath the dura mater. This type of hemorrhage can result from a punch just under the jaw.

An intracerebral hemorrhage is bleeding within the brain. This injury commonly occurs in the frontal and temporal lobes. Severe impact injury can cause both contusions on the brain surface and bleeding within the brain. Impacts of great force, such as car accidents, are common causes of intracerebral hemorrhages. Because blood is irritating to the brain, intracerebral hemorrhage can cause seizures.

Pressure on the Brain

Any form of bleeding either outside or within the brain can increase the pressure in the brain. In an epidural hematoma, blood can quickly expand and collect, pressing on the brain and increasing the pressure within it. Such increased pressure can become a serious problem because the skull normally protects the brain by keeping it within the skull's bony "cage" and because the brain fills most of the space within this cage. Additional pressure on the brain, however, forces the brain to move somewhere. Elevated pressure can push the brain into the major opening of the skull, a hole through which the spine connects to the brain. The diameter of this hole is much smaller than the brain, so any part of the brain driven into this hole is essentially strangled, resulting in a condition called herniation. Herniation of this type can lead to death because it damages the brainstem areas that control breathing.

Blast injuries are now more prevalent in American military personnel due to the recent wars in the Middle East and Afghanistan. The exact nature of brain injuries after a blast explosion is unknown, but research suggests that the gear soldiers wear to protect the torso forces the pressure from the blast up to the head, causing brain injuries.

Oxygen Deprivation

As we noted above, the consequences of penetrating TBI include not only direct damage to brain tissue but also bleeding in the brain. Bleeding in the brain can have consequences beyond just increased pressure; bleeding can endanger the brain's oxygen supply. Red blood cells in the bloodstream carry oxygen molecules, so a bleeding blood vessel reduces the oxygen supply to the brain. The result is called an anoxic (absence of oxygen) injury. Anoxic injury can also lead to inflammation, which in turn can lead to the death of brain cells. People who survive a penetrating brain injury are prone to developing seizures.

Damage to Neurons

Trauma to the brain can cause injury to the neurons and also injury to the axons, all of which can interfere with normal brain functioning. Figure 3.2 shows common types of brain cell injury that occur in a TBI. Axons are connecting fibers between neurons and form the white matter tissue of the brain. The back-and-forth movement of the soft brain within the bony skull during trauma can stretch and tear the axons, a condition known as diffuse axonal injury (DAI). These TBIs occur in inertial injuries, particularly those occurring in car accidents in which the head is not hit, but the brain moves within the skull. If severe enough, DAI can lead to coma and

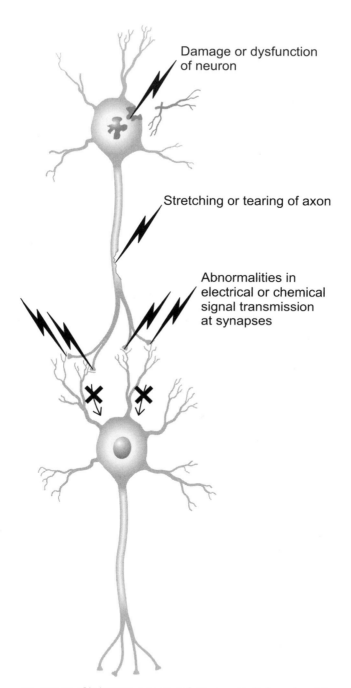

Damage or dysfunction of neuron

Stretching or tearing of axon

Abnormalities in electrical or chemical signal transmission at synapses

Figure 3.2. Types of injury to neurons that can result from head trauma

death—if the axons stretch so hard or so far that they snap and detach from the neuron. Mild TBIs can result from diffuse axonal injuries even if damage does not appear on brain imaging studies, such as computerized tomography (CT) or magnetic resonance imaging (MRI) scans. A new form of brain scan called diffusion tensor imaging (DTI) is better than CT or MRI at detecting axonal injuries. DTI and other new scanning techniques are mainly research tools at present, but they may be used in the future to evaluate patients for DAI.

In this chapter, we reviewed the major types and mechanics of TBI and bleeding within and outside of the brain. Brain bleeds are life-threatening conditions requiring immediate medical care. Consult with a medical professional at the first sign of new or abnormal symptoms after head trauma, such as headache, dizziness, confusion, disorientation, or fogginess. Other common symptoms of brain bleeds are loss of consciousness, sudden severe headache, seizures, vomiting, weakness in the arms or legs, difficulty speaking, or sudden changes in vision.

In the next chapter, we build upon the knowledge we have gained and discuss how the brain can recover from the various types of injuries we discussed. We focus on the notion of brain plasticity, that is, the dynamic nature of the brain. The brain is able to change, and indeed, it is changing all the time as it processes and learns new information. We discuss how this notion is relevant to recovery from TBI.

4

Influences on Recovery after Traumatic Brain Injury

On a foggy October morning, 67-year-old Wilson was involved in a multivehicle crash on a country road. He was driving the fourth of five vehicles in the accident chain. The fifth car plowed into the back of Wilson's car at about 50 mph, driving his car into and under the car in front of him. Wilson sustained cuts and bruises to his face. He apparently never lost consciousness, but the Emergency Medical Services team found him dazed and disoriented at the scene of the accident, so they transported him to the local emergency department for evaluation. The results of a computerized tomography (CT) scan of his head and neck were normal. Wilson was diagnosed with concussion and discharged that afternoon.

The day after the accident Wilson felt pain in his neck, back, and head. He saw an orthopedic physician, who diagnosed him with whiplash injury. Several days later, Wilson saw a neurologist because he was having difficulty focusing, couldn't think clearly, had headaches, couldn't sleep, and felt anxious. His neurological exam was normal, as was a brain magnetic resonance imaging (MRI) scan. Wilson took several cognitive tests about a week after the accident and performed poorly on tests of processing speed and verbal memory. The neurologist determined that the sleep problems, headaches, and anxiety resulted from the concussion and recommended Tylenol (acetaminophen) as needed for the headaches. He educated

Wilson about concussions and sleep hygiene and suggested his patient take another week off from work. He did not prescribe any medications.

Over the next two months, Wilson's symptoms gradually improved. He repeated the cognitive tests about two months after the accident and showed improvement on tests of information processing and verbal memory. According to his wife, he was "functioning as usual" about eight weeks after the accident.

WE EXAMINED BRAIN STRUCTURE AND FUNCTION in some detail in earlier chapters. We described different types of traumatic brain injury in Chapter 3. In this chapter, we attempt to explain how the brain can recover from injury of various types. We think that knowing how the brain recovers will help you understand the discussions of psychiatric symptoms of TBI starting in the next chapter, because the behavioral interventions we suggest are based at least in part on brain recovery principles.

The brain is dynamic by nature, as it must be to make sense of a dynamic, changing world. There is inherent plasticity to the brain— that is, the brain can learn new ways of doing old things. This characteristic can help the brain recover from injury, as it enables us to train the brain using rehabilitation techniques.

The extent of recovery after TBI depends on the severity of the injury. In cases of mild TBI, recovery within a few months is the rule, although a small percentage of people experience persistent symptoms. In cases of moderate to severe brain injury, recovery may be slower and often depends on rehabilitation and support from family and friends. In this chapter, we discuss brain recovery in the context of TBIs of different severities. We start with recovery after mild TBI and discuss recovery from severe TBI later in the chapter.

After a mild TBI (also known as a concussion), people can experience physical symptoms (including dizziness, headaches, sensitivity to light or sound), cognitive symptoms (usually problems with attention or memory), and mood symptoms (irritability, depression, anxiety). People who have these symptoms may feel that they will never improve. The good news is that most people do in fact get better. Many people improve within a month, more by three months, and most by a year. Wilson's recovery, in our opening story, is fairly typical of recovery from mild TBI.

Of course, the rate of recovery varies from person to person, and certain types of symptom improve more quickly than others. People will be more vulnerable to dizziness, for example, if the TBI affects the inner ear. Others may be more vulnerable to cognitive symptoms, such as inattention and slowed thinking. Some people who have many symptoms recover very quickly (within days), whereas for others it may take months to recover fully. Still others have persistent symptoms after mild TBI.

Why this variability in recovery? The exact nature of the injury plays a role, of course, but certain conditions affecting the person either before or after a mild TBI can significantly affect his or her recovery.

Conditions before a Mild TBI
Emotional State

Factors in place before the injury may play a role in determining a person's emotional state after a TBI. Preexisting mood or emotional disturbances can be a factor, so let's use anxiety as an example. If a person who suffers from anxiety suffers a mild TBI, he is at increased risk of becoming more anxious after the TBI. Anxiety can increase because of the stress of suffering the TBI or because the TBI affected areas of the brain that control anxiety. The increase in anxiety can be obvious, making the sufferer feel more anxious, but it can also manifest in physical ways. The person with TBI may be more sensitive to physical signals—slight dizziness or brief twinges of pain—that he might have ignored before his accident. He may have trouble concentrating and thus have problems with memory. These symptoms may be part of the TBI, but anxiety can also cause them.

Mood problems that were present before a mild TBI, like depression, can also affect the manifestation of symptoms after TBI. Depression can appear as slowness in thinking or problems with attention or memory, all of which could just as well be due to the TBI. Depression, like anxiety, can worsen after mild TBI. If depression (and anxiety) remain untreated after the TBI, then recovery from symptoms ascribed to TBI can be slow.

Depression may not only cause confusion as to what is due to the TBI and what is due to other factors but it may also directly impact recovery. For example, the person with depression may be less likely to follow up on rehabilitation or engage in behaviors, like exercise, that can facilitate recovery. Evidence from other neuropsychiatric conditions shows that depression may directly affect how the brain recovers. So getting treatment for mood and anxiety symptoms after a TBI will improve quality of life and may also improve recovery.

Drug and Alcohol Use

Another factor that can impact recovery from symptoms after TBI is substance and alcohol use. Alcohol and other mind-altering substances (for example, cocaine, heroin, and marijuana) can directly impair the brain and thus impact recovery. These substances can also worsen mood and anxiety, thereby affecting the manifestation of symptoms. It is critical to avoid such substances to allow optimal recovery. In addition, abuse or misuse of pain pills (Percocet [oxycodone/acetaminophen] or Vicodin [hydrocodone/acetaminophen], for example) or tranquilizers (Valium [diazepam], Xanax [alprazolam], Ativan [lorazepam]) is not only dangerous but can also interfere with recovery.

Overall Personality

Personality factors can also play a role in recovery after mild TBI. Prominent anxiety traits may color how persons with TBI perceive their improvement. In other words, even if an anxious person with TBI is improving as expected, he may not be satisfied with his progress. Such thinking can prolong symptoms. Those with lifelong mood instability likewise can react catastrophically to a mild TBI. Conversely, those who accept the mild TBI as something that, while unfortunate, is not a catastrophe, may recover more quickly.

Previous TBIs

We now believe that the number of previous TBIs can impact recovery. It may be harder to recover from the fourth TBI than the first. Chronic traumatic encephalopathy (CTE) is a recently coined name for the developing concept that accumulated damage from a series of even mild TBIs may lead to long-term impairment over the years. The few available studies suggest that CTE can manifest as behavioral or cognitive problems, with depression or dementia, and at autopsy, the brain shows characteristic physical damage. There is still a lot we don't know about CTE—why some people with multiple mild TBIs develop CTE and others do not. But it is clear that multiple TBIs are not good for the brain, and having a history of multiple TBIs can adversely impact recovery.

Conditions after a Mild TBI

Several critical factors after a mild TBI will affect recovery: social support, the person's availability and willingness to change his lifestyle to improve recovery, emotional state (including posttraumatic stress disorder), and litigation and legal compensation issues. Lifestyle issues can affect recovery after a mild TBI. Although it is important to rest and not engage in athletic activity after a mild TBI until cleared by a doctor, once cleared, exercise may help in various ways. Exercise may improve mood, which in turn may alleviate TBI symptoms. But it is important to develop a recovery plan based on the doctors' recommendations.

Supportive Social Network

Social support is an important factor in recovery. Although this may seem obvious, it is borne out by clinical experience and studies. Having a strong social network and family support can allow more time for rest, which is critical for optimal recovery. Emotional support from friends, family, and medical personnel may also directly affect the brain's ability to recover in ways that we don't yet understand.

If a person with TBI has had psychological trauma in the past, whether physical, emotional, or sexual abuse, an important aspect of recovery is how that person integrates the TBI into his self-concept. Thinking about the TBI less catastrophically may help with recovery. Being willing and able to participate in psychotherapy can help the person integrate the TBI into his life story. Talking it out with family and friends can help with this, too. Practicing meditative and yoga techniques after TBI may also be helpful in this process.

Emotional State

Mood and anxiety symptoms that develop after mild TBI can clearly impact recovery. In particular, posttraumatic stress disorder (PTSD) may develop after mild TBI. The core symptoms of PTSD are re-experiencing the trauma (in nightmares or flashbacks), being on edge (being easily startled or irritable), and avoiding thinking about the trauma. PTSD may complicate recovery from symptoms after a TBI, especially if the PTSD symptoms are not addressed directly. PTSD symptoms can be hard to distinguish from mild TBI symptoms because some symptoms overlap, but clinicians with expertise in this area can manage the condition appropriately.

Legal Issues

Litigation and compensation factors are controversial issues in recovery after mild TBI. There will always be those who abuse the system and try to get compensation after a mild TBI by exaggerating symptoms. But there are others who truly have symptoms after a mild TBI. Sometimes symptoms may not be the direct result of TBI but may be associated with the frustration and stress of dealing with the legal system, the police, or insurance companies.

Recovery after Moderate to Severe TBI

Recovery after a moderate to severe TBI depends on a number of factors. Both the medical treatment received soon after the injury and the amount of brain tissue damage incurred affect the quality and success of recovery from severe TBI. In most cases, immediate and appropriate medical or surgical treatment for conditions such as brain swelling or bleeding in the brain will increase the likelihood of a successful recovery. Similarly, the less damage to brain tissue, the greater the chance for recovery over time.

Rehabilitation plays a particularly large role in the immediate treatment of significant TBI. Substantial physical, occupational, or cognitive rehabilitation is often necessary. The quality of this rehabilitation, and the patient's ability and willingness to undergo the rehabilitation, can affect recovery.

Of course, the severity of the TBI is an important influence on recovery. The outlook is poor for those who are in a vegetative state after TBI, meaning that they have lost meaningful cognitive function and awareness but continue breathing on their own.

Even among those with severe TBI who are not in a vegetative state, long-term cognitive problems can impact recovery. There is some evidence that moderate to severe TBI increases one's risk for developing Alzheimer's dementia and Parkinson's disease, although not all studies support this.

As with mild TBI, emerging mood, anxiety, and personality issues can affect optimal recovery after severe TBI. Family and friends of a person who has had severe TBI must acknowledge that their loved one may never get back to the way he was prior to the TBI. Accepting this "new baseline" can help the person integrate the TBI into his sense of self. If he recovers only partially, the challenge is to help him achieve the best quality of life possible given his new circumstances. Psychotherapy and lifestyle practices like meditation can be effective tools in adjusting to "the new normal."

In this chapter, we covered a number of factors that affect recovery after TBI. It certainly makes sense that persons with mild TBI are more likely to recover fully, and faster, than those with moderate to severe TBI. Support from family and friends is important no matter what the severity of the TBI. Help your loved one obtain appropriate medical care, rehabilitation, psychotherapy if needed, and treatment for chronic mood and anxiety disorders. Family, friends, and caretakers of someone with TBI play a critical role in helping the person make sense of the trauma, both physical and psychological, accept what has happened, and consequently recover.

PART II

Emotional Problems Caused by the Traumatized Brain

In Part One, we discussed the structure and function of the brain and aspects of brain recovery. In Part Two, we delve into specific psychiatric symptoms after TBI. We focus on emotional or mood problems that can occur and persist after TBI. These symptoms, such as depression or mania, can significantly impact quality of life and recovery from the brain injury. It is often difficult for family and friends to understand that these symptoms can occur as a direct result of TBI, because people may think mood changes are a natural reaction to injury or the loss associated with the injury. This may well be a factor, but injury to the brain can also create disturbances in brain chemicals that can contribute to mood changes. Emotional problems after TBI quite commonly arise. In this section, we explore depression, mania, anxiety, and apathy (lack of motivation).

5

Depression

At 33, John was a successful carpenter working on a construction site when he fell from a ladder 40 feet to the ground. When he didn't regain consciousness after the fall, his co-workers called an ambulance, which sped him to the nearest hospital. Brain scans revealed that John was bleeding in the right and left frontal lobes and the left temporal lobe. He remained in a coma in the intensive care unit for two weeks. His doctors monitored his brain swelling and vital signs and decided against performing brain surgery because the bleeding was gradually resolving.

Three weeks after his fall, John was alert and gradually regaining his ability to care for himself. He could mostly feed himself, go to the bathroom, and get dressed with little help from the hospital staff. He was transferred to an inpatient rehabilitation unit, where he received speech and language therapy, physical therapy, and occupational therapy. After a month of rehabilitation, he was better able to get around on his own and independently take care of his personal hygiene and grooming. John was discharged home and continued to receive outpatient occupational, physical, and speech and language therapy for the next six months.

Soon after John came home, his family and friends noticed that he was just not the same person he had been before the injury. He was often sad, and he cried frequently. John disengaged from his family and friends and kept to himself in his bedroom. If he spoke to other people, it was only to apologize for being "useless and worthless." He said he "didn't deserve to live" and would be "better off dead."

John's periods of sadness lasted for two or three weeks at a time. During these episodes, he didn't eat much, slept poorly, and said he was always tired. He tried to go back to work a few times, but just couldn't keep up. "I just feel numb," he said. Eventually John's boss had to let him go because his poor performance was endangering the other workers. Once he lost his job, John distanced himself even further from his wife and children, and his wife eventually left him, taking the children with her. Only after his family came apart did John ask his doctor for help, explaining that he had completely lost interest in life and could no longer go on.

THE WORD DEPRESSION HAS BECOME common in daily conversation. We say we are depressed over a bad relationship, or a bad job situation, or even a bad day. When people use the word *depression* in this way, they don't mean clinical depression. People use *depression* and *depressed* to describe feeling sad about something that would cause most people to feel sad. If we don't get the promotion we think we deserve, or if we get into a fight with our spouse, or if our child gets into trouble in school, we may call it *being depressed*, but what we really are feeling is appropriate sadness. Sadness is not pathological. Sadness is a normal human emotion.

Clinical depression, also known as major depression, on the other hand, is a medical diagnosis describing sustained, persistent low (depressed) mood in a person who cannot enjoy usual activities and who may have physical symptoms such as trouble with sleep and concentration.

Unfortunately, inaccurate use of this medical term has permeated popular culture, making it harder for people to understand what depression really is. Our use of the word in this way makes it seem as if depression is not really a medical problem, but rather a "normal" response to life's setbacks. Yet clinical depression is a medical condition and not a normal response to events.

Further complicating the situation is that, even in a medical sense, depression is not a single concept. Depression comes in many forms and has many diagnoses: major depressive disorder, dysthymia, bipolar depression, depressive disorder not otherwise specified, adjustment disorder with depressed mood, and many others. Depression is thus a spectrum of disorders, all of which can affect people mildly or severely, ranging from minor effects on relationships and work to suicide.

What separates a diagnosis of clinical depression from normal sadness—what separates pathology from normality—is whether the symptoms significantly affect functioning. Clinical depression can affect work performance, social relationships, home life, or any combination of these. Furthermore, to warrant the diagnosis of clinical depression, functioning must be persistently affected for a minimum amount of time (at least two weeks for a diagnosis of major depression). Clinical depression is not an afternoon spent mourning or "having the blues" over a troubling situation. Clinical depression, in fact, can be autonomous, that is, unrelated to any single troubling event. It may occur with no "good reason" and persist for weeks or months. Of course, those who have had a TBI, and their family members, may already know from their own experience what major depression is, but using the correct terminology for it affects how people perceive what depressed patients are struggling with.

Symptoms

In traumatic brain injury, depressive symptoms are rather common, but here we have to be even more careful with terminology, because these symptoms may not fit neatly into a category such as major depressive disorder. Depression in TBI may be more diffuse and hard to diagnose precisely. Many factors can cause clinical depression after TBI: having a history of major depression before the TBI (a well-known risk factor), the severity of the injury (more severe injury increasing the risk), alcohol or substance abuse, and the presence of psychosocial problems (for example, minimal emotional support, poor finances, unemployment) before and after TBI. How exactly TBI causes major depression is unclear. TBI can act as a stressor and cause depression in someone who is already vulnerable to depression, or it can cause dysfunction of neural circuits or neurochemicals and trigger depression. Most TBI researchers believe that it probably does both.

Unfortunately, persons with TBI or their family members may be told by well-meaning people that it is "understandable" that they are depressed: "Of course you're depressed! Look what you just went through." Even medical professionals may succumb to this fallacy of thinking. It is not unusual to hear nonpsychiatric physicians say such things to their TBI patients. But, as we have discussed, it is not normal for a person with TBI to be depressed—that is, clinically depressed, in the medical sense of the word. Depression is common in TBI, but it is not necessary. *Clinical depression is not a normal part of recovery from brain injury.*

This is an important distinction. When friends, or family, or even medical personnel accept depression as normal after TBI, they are doing the patient a disservice. The subtle implication is that these symptoms do not deserve treatment; after all, if this is normal, why treat it? And what may be implied when depressive symptoms persist is that the patient should be "getting over it." So the person with TBI can interpret this attitude to mean that he has a character flaw or some kind of personal weakness. This message, of course, can make the patient feel even worse, thus perpetuating a cycle of deepening depression.

Consider John, in our opening story. His sadness was associated with a number of prolonged, pervasive, and disruptive physical and emotional symptoms. His is a classic example of major depression, also known as clinical depression: a state of persistent sadness or persistent lack of enjoyment often associated with feelings of hopelessness, low self-worth or guilt, and suicidal thoughts. Other symptoms of major depression are changes in sleep, appetite, energy, or concentration, but because these symptoms are also common consequences of the injury to the brain, medical evaluation is necessary to determine whether a person with these symptoms has major depression. Depressive symptoms persist for consecutive days, disrupt the person's life, and interfere with the person's day-to-day functioning. The rate of suicide in people with depression is about

15 percent. Severe major depression can be associated with hallucinations (hearing, seeing, feeling, or smelling things when there are no external stimuli) or delusions (fixed, false beliefs), or both.

Major depression can interfere with recovery from a brain injury; people with major depression may not recover as well from the TBI as those without depression. TBI survivors who suffer from major depression show greater impairment in their ability to function, and they have poorer outcomes than TBI survivors who are not depressed. Depression after TBI can also be associated with alcohol and drug use, which in turn can impair recovery. Alcohol toxicity and TBI may have a synergistic effect and produce more severe structural brain damage and affect chemical pathways in the brain. Persons with major depressive disorder after TBI are more likely to be irritable, act aggressively, and be anxious.

Conditions That Mimic Major Depression

We have discussed how clinical depression is different from normal sadness. However, to complicate matters further, several other disorders may look like major depression, but be quite different.

One possibility to consider when a person appears depressed is that the person has bipolar depression. We discuss bipolar disorder in more detail in Chapter 7 ("Mania"), but we mention it here because depression, along with mania, is part of bipolar disorder. Depression as part of bipolar disorder can be hard, even for experts, to distinguish from major depression, but there are some clues. Bipolar depression may begin earlier in life than major depression and have more mood variability, that is, more exaggerated response to stress. The person with bipolar depression may eat more and sleep more (as opposed to eating less and sleeping less, traits more typical in major depression). These are all clues to the possibility of bipolar depression, but the one clear way to distinguish between bipolar depression and major depression is that in bipolar depression, these periods of depression alternate with periods of heightened energy, mood, and activity (mania). The treatment for bipolar depression is quite different from the treatment for major depression, so a correct diagnosis is important.

Another possibility to keep in mind when a person appears depressed is a condition called pseudobulbar affect (PBA), also known as pathological laughing and crying, or emotional incontinence. PBA is fairly common in TBI, especially in moderate to severe injuries. A person with PBA can cry or laugh for no apparent reason or cry or laugh excessively in relation to what they are reacting to. In other words, someone with PBA may see something on TV that is a bit sad and begin to cry excessively and be unable to stop. Or the person with PBA may not actually feel sad when he is crying; he might be crying for no good reason and not, in truth, be sad at all. The cause of PBA is still not clear. While some believe that it is due to lack of control of emotions due to damage to brain circuits that normally keep emotions in check, others believe that it is related to difficulty with facial expressions, and so crying or laughing can occur without being accompanied by sadness or happiness. Absence of persistent low mood is a key point that differentiates pathological crying of PBA from major depression. Major depression is a mood disorder, and the person suffering from it experiences relentless sadness. In contrast, in pathological crying of PBA, there is tearfulness in the absence of sadness or disproportionate to the sadness felt. Treatment for PBA may be different from treatment for major depression.

Brain Circuits Affected by Depression

Clinical depression clearly has a neurobiological basis. We have a fairly good idea at this point what parts of the brain are involved in generating symptoms of depression (figure 5.1). An evolutionarily primitive core area deep within the brain known as the limbic system is involved in generating emotions. The limbic system borders the cortex, the part of the brain involved in thinking and planning.

Parts of the limbic system, including the hippocampus, the amygdala, and the anterior cingulate, are probably involved in the genesis of clinical depression. In fact, an area of the anterior cingulate called the subgenual cingulate may be a key region associated with depression. Current thinking (or at least a popular theory) is that increased activity in the subgenual cingulate may be associated with depression. The subgenual cingulate is a key part of the neural

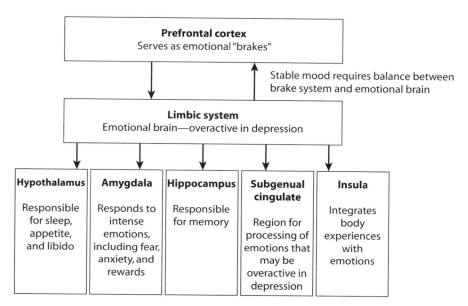

Figure 5.1. Regions of the brain associated with depression

circuit that connects the frontal lobe cortex (the thinking and planning part of the brain) to the limbic system, the emotional brain. The frontal lobe cortex normally acts as a "brake" to prevent the subgenual cingulate from getting hyperactive. If this "brake" fails, the subgenual cingulate is free to become hyperactive, leading to increased emotional discharge—in other words, depression.

Clinical depression can occur without directly affecting the limbic system deep within the brain. Damage to the frontal lobe cortex (which, as we've noted, is highly vulnerable to trauma) can result in depression by removing this "brake" and allowing the limbic system to be hyperactive and letting the "emotional brain" dominate the "thinking and planning brain."

Of course, it is possible for brain trauma to directly affect the limbic system as well, despite its location deep within the brain. The hippocampus portion of the limbic system can shrink in major depression, and shrinkage can be even more pronounced in those who have both TBI and major depression.

There may be other ways that affecting circuits in the brain, directly or indirectly, leads to increased clinical depression. The key concept, however, is that anything that disturbs the balance between the "emotional brain" and the "thinking and planning brain" by making the former more dominant may cause depressive symptoms.

Evidence also suggests that the left frontal cortex in particular is involved in depression. People who have had left frontal cortex strokes are prone to depression. The left hemisphere of the brain (which houses much of our language abilities) may act as a storyteller of our lives, and this may decrease the risk of depression by weaving together the tapestry of our life events that may otherwise have been depressing into a coherent and understandable story. But damage to the left hemisphere may prevent it from creating a story out of life events in an appropriate way, and so may increase the risk of depression.

Treatment

Treating depression is important because depression can have biological effects. Research data suggest that depression is associated with inflammation in the body. Depression can increase the levels of stress hormones such as cortisol or increase adrenaline and impair the immune system. These changes can increase the risk for certain medical illnesses, including heart disease and arthritis. We know that depression contributes to worse outcomes in people who have had heart attacks or who have diabetes or Alzheimer's disease.

Regardless of the cause, be it the brain injury itself or poor social support, depression has a detrimental effect on the brain. Clinical depression can make patients engage in unsafe behaviors like using drugs or alcohol. People who are clinically depressed may not participate in rehabilitation as they otherwise would; many ignore their health, eat poorly, and don't exercise.

What can you do if you think you or someone you know and care for is clinically depressed after brain injury? Get professional help! Only professionals can differentiate among the many faces of depression. Getting an accurate diagnosis from a professional is crucial because treatment differs for different conditions. Major depression and similar conditions are often treated with a combination of medication and counseling or psychotherapy.

Drug Therapy

Many medications are available to treat depression; all are more or less equally effective, but each has different side effects. People with TBI may be more sensitive than people without TBI to certain medications. Neuropsychiatrists (doctors who are trained in psychiatry and who have experience treating mood, behavioral, and cognitive symptoms in neurologic disorders like TBI) will choose the most appropriate medications. General psychiatrists, neurologists, physiatrists, and primary care doctors also often treat these symptoms. The medication choice depends on the person's emotional and behavioral problems, medical issues, other medications the person is taking, and the person's family medical history. No one should take a medication or adjust the dose of a medication or stop a medication without first getting his doctor's advice.

You may be familiar with the concept that depression is related to a "chemical imbalance" in the brain resulting from too little serotonin. Serotonin is clearly part of the story of depression. Studies show that people who were depressed and impulsively committed suicide had very low levels of serotonin. Medications for depression, such as selective serotonin reuptake inhibitors (SSRIs), are believed to increase serotonin, thus alleviating depression. The success of SSRIs in treating depression has validated the important role of serotonin in depression. SSRIs are the mainstay of depression treatment today. Most doctors prefer to treat major depression using SSRIs because of their mild side effects. Common medications in this family include Celexa (citalopram), Zoloft (sertraline), Lexapro (escitalopram), and Prozac (fluoxetine).

The circuitry that we have discussed in this chapter is associated with a significant number of serotonin receptors; there thus may be a connection between serotonin (part of what we call a chemical model of depression) and the subgenual cingulate (part of an anatomical model of depression), as serotonin may play a prominent role in areas of the brain important for mood regulation.

Other chemicals likely involved in depression are norepinephrine and dopamine. Norepinephrine and dopamine may be important in attention and motivation. Many people with depression have problems concentrating and focusing and have trouble getting motivated to do what they know they need to do. Such problems are common after TBI, and depression can worsen these symptoms. Medications known as serotonin-norepinephrine reuptake inhibitors (SNRIs) increase norepinephrine and serotonin levels and help depression. Examples of SNRIs are medications like Effexor (venlafaxine), Pristiq (desvenlafaxine), and Fetzima (levomilnacipran). Wellbutrin (bupropion) increases dopamine levels predominantly.

The chemical and anatomical models are likely both correct; they just explain depression at two different levels. Of course, this being the brain, things may be more complicated than that. Despite their names, SSRIs and SNRIs don't merely increase serotonin and alleviate depression. If they did, SSRIs and SNRIs would work very quickly, within hours or days. They don't. They take weeks to work, and here's why: SSRIs and other antidepressants stimulate physical remodeling of the brain. That is, they cause brain circuits to grow and change. This takes weeks, and the mechanism of remodeling, which takes time, explains the few weeks' lag between when a person begins taking antidepressants and when he feels their full effects.

This remodeling process ties in with our earlier discussion of inflammation. Levels of certain hormones called growth factors may increase when a person is taking SSRIs. These increased growth factor levels stimulate growth in brain circuits. Inflammation may impair these growth factors.

In discussing neuronal circuits and neurochemistry we do not mean to suggest that there is no psychosocial component to depression. There certainly is. Clearly, poor support from family, an unstable living situation, or a stressful work environment can worsen mood in people who have depression. These psychosocial factors, however, also work by means of some of the same mechanisms in the brain as the brain injury itself. That is, psychosocial factors may worsen depression by affecting some of the same circuits, via serotonin, and by affecting growth factors. They may cause emotional hyperreactivity in the limbic system. They may cause "faulty thoughts" in the frontal cortex, allowing the emotional brain to dominate behavior.

In other words, some people are particularly vulnerable to life stressors because they have abnormal levels of serotonin, norepinephrine, or dopamine. When they have a major life stressor such as a TBI, they are prone to an increase in inflammatory chemicals, which can lead to an increase of cortisol, which is a stress hormone. This increase in cortisol can lead to shrinkage of the hippocampus and to an imbalance between the emotional brain and the thinking brain. The thinking brain cannot curb the overactive emotional brain, and the result is emotional instability.

We have discussed medications like SSRIs for depression. The discussion has so far focused on major depression. However, as we discussed earlier, bipolar depression may be an explanation for depressive symptoms rather than major depression. The treatment for bipolar depression is quite different, and in fact, if someone has bipolar disorder and is put on an SSRI only, there is the possibility that symptoms overall could get worse. Bipolar disorder often needs a mood stabilizer like Depakote (valproic acid), lithium, Lamictal (lamotrigine), or Tegretol (carbamazepine). Oftentimes, another agent is necessary. Seroquel (quetiapine) and Latuda (lurasidone) are approved by the Food and Drug Administration (FDA) for acute treatment of bipolar depression.

Pseudobulbar affect (PBA) may potentially be treated with SSRI medications. Nuedexta (dextromethorphan/quinidine) is a medication approved by the FDA for treating PBA in neurological conditions, with evidence from multiple sclerosis and amyotrophic lateral sclerosis (ALS, or Lou Gehrig's disease) patients in particular. Nuedexta specifically reduces the symptoms of PBA only; it does not treat depression. It is not yet entirely clear if PBA symptoms in TBI would respond to Nuedexta as they do in multiple sclerosis or ALS.

Neuromodulation Therapy

Neuromodulation therapy is therapy that alters or modulates parts of the brain directly using forces such as electricity or magnetism. Repeated application of these forces to parts of the brain over time can cause changes in the way neurons in those parts of the brain interact. The importance of appreciating brain circuitry is that new neuromodulation techniques for treating clinical depression may directly or indirectly affect parts of the brain circuits associated with depression.

Deep brain stimulation is a technique in which electrodes are implanted in the subgenual cingulate and other regions of the brain. When activated, these electrodes act as a "pacemaker" for the brain, activating the frontal cortex and deactivating the subgenual cingulate.

Transcranial magnetic stimulation (TMS) is another technique that uses an electromagnetic coil, which is placed over the scalp and focused on an area of the brain thought to be involved in mood regulation. The coil generates brief magnetic pulses, which pass through the bony skull into the brain and stimulates brain cells involved in maintaining emotional balance. These pulses are administered in rapid succession. Activating the frontal cortex with this device does ameliorate depression; TMS is an FDA-approved treatment for major depression in the general population. There are currently ongoing studies to determine the effectiveness of TMS in persons with TBI and depression.

Additional treatment techniques currently under study are magnetic seizure therapy, in which a magnetic field is used to induce seizures that may help depression, and transient direct current stimulation, in which a weak electrical current is applied to the brain. Electroconvulsive therapy (ECT), or shock therapy, has been around for decades and successive improvements over the years have made the therapy more tolerable and more focused. ECT remains a treatment of choice for severe depression.

Psychotherapy

Psychotherapy (or talk therapy) is a form of treatment that aims to teach skills and approaches to better understand and manage emotional reactions. In psychotherapy, the person learns techniques for coping with stressful circumstances and negative thoughts. All forms of depression respond well to psychotherapy in combination with appropriate antidepressant medications (when needed). A mental health professional can choose the type and the duration of psychotherapy that is best for each person. Psychologists (who have PhD degrees), mental health therapists, and clinical social workers (who have LCSW certification or MSW degrees) can do therapy. Most forms of talk therapy are short-term, focused, and specific in their approach.

The goal of supportive therapy is to provide hope and to educate about the illness or the circumstances associated with stress and depression. Supportive therapy in the case of TBI could include discussing how the TBI has affected the person's outlook and family. The therapist can provide concrete suggestions about how best to adjust to the new life situation the person with TBI is facing.

Cognitive behavioral therapy (CBT) is based on the principle that thoughts and feelings influence a person's behavior. Thoughts can lead to certain feelings, which in turn can lead to behaviors. The concept of CBT is to train someone to think more like a scientist, to examine whether the thoughts he is having are valid or supported by evidence. A person who has depression may have thoughts pop into his mind that are not supported by evidence (for example, "I will never get better" or "It's no use" or "No one likes me"). In CBT, the patient learns not to accept any thoughts that come into his mind without examining them and being skeptical of their validity.

Therapists trained in CBT teach their patients to recognize negative thought patterns and to substitute them with more realistic ones. In this way, the person's behavior can be converted to more productive and healthy activities. CBT therapists usually work with patients once a week for a set period of time (for example, 12 weeks). At the end of each session, the therapist may assign homework so that the patient continues to practice working with his thoughts every day as he goes about his life. CBT can also be simply behavior therapy or behavior modification therapy (the behavioral aspect of CBT), the goal being to change abnormal behavior and to help patients unlearn behavior patterns that contribute to their feelings of sadness or make them worse. Behavioral therapies include relaxation training, stress management, biofeedback, desensitization, exposure therapy, and mindfulness meditation.

Personal interactions can be problematic because of the physical and emotional consequences of TBI; depression on top of those conditions can lead to poor communication and an inability to express emotion. The goal of interpersonal therapy (IPT) is to help the person improve interpersonal skills and either resolve or cope with interpersonal problems. IPT focuses on learning effective communication, expressing emotions appropriately, and being appropriately assertive (that is, learning which situations call for assertiveness and how to be assertive when appropriate). IPT can help the person with TBI regain or improve these communication skills.

Dialectical behavioral therapy (DBT) focuses on distressing problematic behaviors and helps the person learn different, more rewarding approaches. The therapist usually focuses on one problematic event at a time and works with the person to understand the events that triggered the behavior. DBT incorporates mindfulness (keeping the mind in the present and accepting one's thoughts and emotions in a nonjudgmental way), a technique often used in cognitive behavioral therapy. DBT teaches skills for regulating emotions and not overreacting to people or events. DBT can be particularly helpful for people who may be overwhelmed by emotions and considering harming themselves.

Family therapy is helpful for people with TBI, and we recommend this as a "must-do" to families who are finding it difficult to adjust and cope after their loved one has had a brain injury. The family therapist brings all the family members together, educates them about brain injury and its consequences, encourages them to acknowledge and talk about the stress in the family (and their relationship with the brain-injured person), and offers strategies to reduce the stress and cope with all the issues raised. Family therapy can incorporate techniques from supportive and cognitive behavioral therapy as well.

In group therapy, a small number of people with similar issues meet regularly (often weekly) with a therapist to discuss their problems and discuss ways of dealing with them. The goal is for patients to learn from one another, with the benefit of professional guidance and feedback from the therapist. It can be hard for people with TBI to find others who understand what they have gone through, what they are feeling now, and the anxieties they have about the future. Sharing concerns, fears, small victories, and coping techniques with others who have experienced similar trauma can be beneficial to people with TBI.

In summary, depression that develops after TBI can be a serious impediment to recovery; it should not be minimized or normalized. If you experience symptoms of clinical depression or notice them in a family member you care for, take quick action to get help. Depression after TBI can result directly from the brain injury itself or indirectly from factors such as loss of a job or an unsupportive family. Depression can make symptoms of the brain injury worse, cause recovery to falter, and contribute to other medical problems. Depression can be a fatal illness. Suicide is not uncommon in people who are clinically depressed. We ignore it at our own and our loved one's peril. If you don't know where to get started in helping yourself or your family member suffering from depression and suicidal thoughts, call your primary care doctor, neurologist, or other trusted professional for suggestions and referrals. Because anxiety and depression often go hand in hand, we discuss anxiety in the next chapter.

Tips for Coping with Depression after TBI

If you are experiencing depression after TBI:

> Organize your day and keep daily timetables. The brain tends to respond well to structure and organization, which may assist with both physical and emotional recovery. If you are unable to do this yourself or are not sure how to go about setting up a schedule, ask your doctor to refer you to a rehabilitation therapist, who can help with daily planning.

> Exercise regularly. Exercise helps with both physical and mental recovery. Exercising for 30 minutes at least three to four times a week is healthy and helpful. Start with a form of exercise you are comfortable with and gradually add other types of exercise. Brisk walking for 20 to 30 minutes is a good place to start. Light weightlifting helps build

strength in the upper body and arms. The key is to exercise consistently.

> Eat healthily. Eating a balanced, nutritional diet across typical waking hours helps maximize brain function and emotional regulation. Do not skip meals. Consult with a nutritionist to learn how to follow a healthy diet. Foods with omega-3 fatty acids (as found in fish oil, algae oil, and flaxseed oil) and B vitamins (such as leafy green vegetables) are good choices to help brain function.

> Exercising your brain by staying active mentally not only helps your brain recover but also helps regulate your emotional state. There is emerging evidence that cognitive exercises (brain training) may help delay the onset of major cognitive problems (like dementia), so it is plausible that such exercises help the brain's ability to "rewire" in TBI. You can keep your brain active just by going about your day-to-day activities such as conversing with others, completing daily life chores, and engaging in pleasurable activities. Puzzles, card games, and board games are cognitive exercises that engage your brain. In general, it is important to keep your brain busy and stay organized.

> Get involved and stay involved with pleasurable activities. Keep it simple and start with what you enjoy most. As you feel comfortable, gradually step up your activities to include more challenging tasks.

> Build in rest breaks. Do not "push through" fatigue. Planning your day to include both active periods and rest periods can maximize your functioning and endurance throughout your day. Rest doesn't necessarily mean napping, but rather low-stimulation activities, like sitting quietly or listening to music. There is no set timetable or rules on how much rest is too much. Use your own body as a "thermometer" to recognize and measure the signs of fatigue.

> Avoid using alcohol and illicit drugs. Continued use of alcohol and other mind-altering drugs can worsen mood states, which is why people with TBI or depression need to abstain

from their use. If you find that you cannot stop using alcohol or drugs on your own, seek professional help.

If you know someone who is experiencing depression after TBI:

> Offer support and understanding. Clinical depression is a *medical condition*, not a sign of weakness or a character flaw. Your consistent support and understanding is valuable to the person recovering from TBI.

> Work with the person to develop a daily timetable that includes time for healthy meals and restful sleep. People with depression tend to have erratic eating and sleeping patterns; they eat and sleep poorly (like John, at the beginning of this chapter) or excessively. Insufficient nutrition or fluid intake (dehydration) can result in a medical emergency requiring hospitalization. Discuss this need for a timetable with the person's physician and request referral to an occupational therapist, who can help with structuring the day.

> Encourage the person to learn and practice sleep hygiene. Healthy sleep habits include going to bed and waking up around the same time every day, using the bed only for sleep and physical intimacy, avoiding caffeinated drinks after 4 p.m., and keeping the bedroom quiet, dim, and relaxing. (For more on sleep hygiene, see "Tips for a Good Night's Sleep" in Chapter 12.)

> Use the buddy system. Social withdrawal and isolation are common in people with depression. Offer to "buddy-up" with your loved one for fun activities or hobbies—exercise together, play checkers, go to the library. However, be prepared for him to want "space"; he may interpret your presence as "being controlling." Use communication strategies that make him feel important and that he is making the decisions. For example, instead of telling your loved one what to do, offer some choices and ask him to pick one: "I want to take a walk. Should we go to the park or the beach?"

> Don't take it personally. People with depression may appear hostile and angry and reject your attempts to provide care.

Conversely, they can become totally dependent on you and shadow you everywhere. Try not to take any of these characteristics personally. Set limits, but balance firmness with gentleness.

If you are concerned about the safety of your family member or friend, call 911 or take the person to the nearest hospital. Self-injurious behavior is not uncommon in depression. Take seriously any comments he may make about suicide and obtain professional help for him.

6

Anxiety

Sara was 43 when she was involved in a serious car accident that resulted in bleeding within her brain. She did well and made gradual progress throughout much of her prolonged hospitalization and eventual rehabilitation. After Sara returned home, however, her husband noticed that she was becoming more and more anxious. She worried excessively about everyday matters. For example, she worried about their children taking the school bus; her concern lasted until they came home. Later in the day, she worried about having dinner ready at the scheduled time or going to bed at her usual time. Her husband also noticed that she worried chronically for no apparent reason about minor things—"this, that, and the other" as he called it. He worried aloud that "She's become a nervous wreck." In addition, Sara was easily distracted, was having trouble falling asleep, and complained of being tired during the day. At first, her husband brushed off these changes as worries related to her accident and hospitalization. But when Sara's anxiety was still problematic after nine months and continued to interfere with her day-to-day functioning, her husband decided to get professional help.

ANXIETY IS COMMON AFTER TBI and can often occur along with depression. Of course, everyone gets anxious to some degree. In fact, there is a very good reason for our brains to have circuits for anxiety. If we were never anxious, even in dangerous situations, we would be tempting fate a lot more! We would be much more likely to put ourselves in danger, and once in danger, not get away quickly enough. Without anxiety our ancestors would have been regular meals for saber-toothed tigers, as they would not have had the sense to get away from these predators.

The anxiety circuits in the brain probably developed as threat detectors. They allow us to scan the environment for threats, and they motivate us to escape from these threats and avoid them in the future. These anxiety circuits, like any other parts of the brain, can sustain damage in a TBI. When they are damaged, patients can develop excess anxiety to the point that it interferes with treatment in the hospital, in rehabilitation, or in their ability to adjust to their normal routines after returning home. These symptoms can create additional friction when family and friends do not realize that the anxiety stems from brain damage.

One of the key parts of the brain involved in anxiety generation is something called the amygdala, which, along with the cortex, gets input from the thalamus. The amygdala is deep within the brain, around the level of the temples. The amygdala senses danger and is part of the memory system of the brain. It is particularly good at remembering threats and is activated when there is a sense of possible threat (along with, to some extent, the insula, another region deep within the brain). When the amygdala senses a threat, it activates other parts of the brain, including the hypothalamus (figure 6.1). The hypothalamus in turn activates the fight-or-flight mechanism by releasing hormones like corticotropin-releasing factor (CRF). CRF acts on the pituitary gland, and adrenocorticotropic hormone (ACTH) is released, which in turn acts on the adrenal glands, situated above our kidneys. The adrenal glands release norepinephrine (also known as noradrenaline), which prepares the body to "fight" or "flee." Blood pressure and blood sugar rise, increasing the supply of energy in our arms and legs to deal with the situation. The heart rate accelerates and breathing rate increases. Combined, all these physical changes can fuel a subjective sense of anxiety.

Damage to anxiety circuits can change people's personalities—instead of becoming more anxious, they might become more impulsive, more risk-prone, and less anxious in situations that they would have avoided before. They can become very different people from

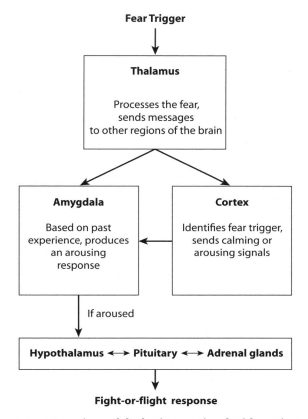

Figure 6.1. Regions of the brain associated with anxiety

who they were before the injury. These personality changes can cause additional problems during treatment and after returning home. Family and friends may not understand why their loved one is so different now, leading to misery on both sides.

Symptoms

Anxiety comes in various forms. Some people with TBI have persistent free-floating anxiety for prolonged periods that interferes with their everyday activities. The medical term for this condition is *generalized anxiety disorder* (GAD). The anxiety symptoms Sara experienced are consistent with GAD. In addition to chronic worry, people with GAD are more on edge and look for danger when there are no obvious reasons for concern. In a sense, their anxiety circuits are overactive. They are perpetually scanning the environment for potential danger. It's like they're looking for the saber-toothed tigers on the plain when in reality there are none. Everyday stresses and strains of life affect people with GAD more than the general population. People with this activated anxiety tend to be more irritable, have trouble with sleep, complain of muscle tension, and feel fatigued. They may realize that they are having trouble controlling how much they worry. As you can see, it can be difficult for family and friends to interact as before with people who develop generalized anxiety disorder after TBI.

If you are involved in the care of a person with TBI who has been suffering from anxiety after the injury, keep in mind that your loved one is not purposely being difficult; being excessively anxious can certainly come out as irritability and impatience, but such behavior doesn't mean that she is targeting you.

Pronounced anxiety can trigger panic attacks—sudden waves of anxiety that occur without warning. A panic attack can be so severe that the person experiencing it sometimes feels that he or she is about to die. Classic symptoms of a panic attack are racing heartbeat, shortness of breath, and a feeling of impending doom. A panic attack is an intense experience and often leads to emergency department visits. Panic attacks can be more prevalent in some people after a brain injury, especially if they were prone to them beforehand.

Anxiety can lead to agitation in some people, especially if they have periods of confusion. This confusion, especially immediately after a severe brain injury, is called delirium. Delirium is an altered state of consciousness somewhere between being awake and being asleep. People experiencing delirium can see things that are not really there (suffer hallucinations) or believe that people, even their doctors or family and friends, are trying to hurt them. In defending themselves against these perceived threats, they can become physically aggressive or agitated. This behavior can be disturbing to family members, who may not understand why their loved one is frightened of them or fighting them. In the hospital, delirious patients may require sedation or, rarely, physical restraint. As disturbing as this can be to family and caregivers, these periods of confusion and high anxiety are temporary. As the brain recovers from the injury, confusion lessens and the anxiety abates.

Anxiety can also manifest as agitation, irritability, frustration, or outbursts of anger in people with TBI who cannot adequately express their emotions. Such bouts of anxiety are usually triggered by actual or perceived stressful situations. For example, simple activities of daily living such as bathing and dressing may be a source of stress and anxiety in persons with severe TBI for a number of reasons: embarrassment about their loss of independence, guilt about having to depend on their loved ones, or resentment that someone is invading their privacy. Anxiety can manifest as frustration or irritability even in those with mild to moderate TBI, when they encounter situations that they could easily have managed before the injury, such as maintaining accounts or planning an event. They may not verbalize their anxiety but express it physically in a flushing face, pacing, fidgeting, muttering, or even screaming.

In some people, anxiety can manifest primarily as general physical symptoms, such as dizziness or headaches. Especially after TBI, whose common aftereffects include dizziness and headaches, it can be difficult to differentiate between what is due to anxiety and what is due to the direct effects of the TBI. In many cases, the two causes coexist: dizziness may come from the TBI but may persist because of the anxiety.

Posttraumatic stress disorder (PTSD) is an anxiety disorder that develops after exposure to a stressful and traumatic event. PTSD can start weeks or months after exposure to the event and last anywhere from a few weeks to several months. During this time, the person re-experiences the trauma in flashbacks or dreams. The person is vigilant and tends to avoid people, places, or situations associated with the traumatic event. With TBI, especially mild TBI, PTSD can co-occur with the brain injury. Soldiers stunned by shrapnel from explosive devices can lose consciousness momentarily and have trouble with memory for several hours, but they may also struggle with mental images of the explosion, the screams of civilians, the smell of sulfur and burning flesh, and guilt about others in their unit dying. These repetitive images, thoughts, and anxieties may become chronic and haunt them for months or years after their tour of duty is over.

It is not unusual for people to become anxious simply because they have had a brain injury and now must adjust to a new way of life. Symptoms of anxiety can also be due to side effects of medications, other medical conditions (e.g., thyroid problems), substance abuse, or withdrawal from drugs such as alcohol, cocaine, or heroin. So if anxiety persists, consult a physician for a thorough evaluation; don't just assume it is attributable to adjustment difficulties after the brain injury.

Treatment
Drug Therapy

Treatment for anxiety after TBI often requires medications. Medications commonly used are selective serotonin reuptake inhibitors (SSRIs) or serotonin-norepinephrine reuptake inhibitors (SNRIs). Commonly used SSRIs include Lexapro (escitalopram), Celexa (citalopram), and Zoloft (sertraline). Effexor (venlafaxine) is a commonly used SNRI. These drugs work well for long-term control of anxiety, but they can take a few weeks to work optimally. The benefit is that they have few major side effects and are not addictive. If SSRIs or SNRIs are ineffective, continue to work with your doctor, because there are other medications that can be used. However, in our opinion, it's best to avoid long-term use of benzodiazepines such as Valium (diazepam), Klonopin (clonazepam), or Ativan (lorazepam) because they can lead to addiction, cause memory problems, and interfere with gait and balance—and may increase agitation.

Psychotherapy

Talk therapy, particularly cognitive behavioral therapy (CBT), is an effective treatment for anxiety, either by itself or in conjunction with medications. To participate in therapy, however, the person with TBI must be able to understand and apply the training, a condition that makes talk therapy a better choice for those with mild to moderate TBI or, for those with severe TBI, after an extensive recovery period.

CBT focuses on understanding the links between feelings and behavior. Typically, the person works with a CBT therapist in regular weekly sessions for a few months. During these sessions the therapist helps the person understand that her maladaptive behavior stems from beliefs that may not be true or realistic or that may be counterproductive. The therapist may assign homework and ask the person to practice behavioral techniques outside the session. The overarching goal is not to focus on an unchangeable external situation but instead to change beliefs or thoughts, which in turn can alter behavior. CBT teaches people to assess the validity of their thoughts and to replace unrealistic thoughts with more valid ones. The anxious person must learn that there are less anxiety-provoking alternative ways to interpret a situation. For example, an anxious person might feel slighted if someone she knows walks by without acknowledging her. CBT would teach her to consider other alternatives, such as, the acquaintance literally may not have seen her or was lost in his or her own thoughts. CBT also teaches anxiety-reducing behavioral techniques such as deep breathing, meditation, creative visualization, and yoga.

In summary, anxiety after TBI can be a significant problem. Some anxiety is healthy, but excessive anxiety can make life miserable and interfere with recovery from TBI. The good news is that there are many treatment options for anxiety. A variety of medications is available to treat anxiety, and talk therapy and lifestyle strategies such as meditation and yoga are often helpful too. A combination of all these techniques may be the best route to resilience and optimal recovery from anxiety after brain injury.

Tips for Coping with Anxiety
If you are experiencing anxiety after TBI:

> ❯ Educate yourself about anxiety symptoms after brain injury. By picking up this book and reading this chapter, you've

taken a big step toward doing that. Read other books or talk to a professional if you are having trouble making sense of your anxiety symptoms. You may feel that these symptoms will never go away; we assure you that anxiety is a treatable condition.

> Consult a professional if anxiety symptoms are persistent or distressing. Contact a psychiatrist, clinical psychologist, or a psychotherapist for help. Any one of these clinicians can refer you to another clinician if you need more help than he or she can provide. For example, if you need medications, a psychologist or psychotherapist can refer you to a psychiatrist who can prescribe an appropriate medication for you.

> Follow the doctor's recommendations and take medications as prescribed. Anxiety symptoms can suddenly worsen. Do not change your dosage on your own or self-medicate if this happens. Talk with your doctor.

> Practice breathing exercises, specifically, abdominal or diaphragmatic breathing. You can learn these techniques from an anxiety coach or therapist, and practice regularly.

If you know someone who is experiencing anxiety after TBI:

> Don't take it personally. As a family member or caregiver, you may encounter some resistance to your well-meaning help and advice. Try not to be upset by the persistent anxiety, and don't take it personally when your loved one gets irritable or edgy.

> Be aware of topics that trigger anxiety. It is important for the person with anxiety to talk about these triggers with a professional and get help. If you are a caregiver, you may not want to bring up a sensitive issue. If the affected person brings it up, listen to her.

> Practice deep breathing and other calming activities, such as meditation or yoga, with your loved one to show your support and caring.

> Make yourself available. Not knowing where to go for help or whom to contact can worsen anxiety. Letting the person with anxiety know that you are only a phone call away can be

reassuring. Encourage her to talk about her anxiety symptoms and listen patiently. Telling her to "buck up" or "get over it" is not helpful; it may be hard for her to disclose her fears if she feels you are judging her.

> Get professional help if you yourself feel overwhelmed, anxious, or irritable in your role as caregiver. It is not uncommon for caregivers to be stressed by their caretaking duties, and it's crucial that you help yourself. After all, only when you are not overwhelmed yourself can you help your family member or friend with anxiety.

7

Mania

Darlene was involved in a serious motor vehicle accident that caused bleeding on the right side of her brain. Her injury required that she be hospitalized for a lengthy period followed by prolonged rehabilitation. Although at 53 Darlene had no history of psychiatric illness, her brother had a history of bipolar disorder, so Darlene's doctors closely monitored her emotional recovery. Her physical symptoms gradually improved, and she remained emotionally stable for about six months.

Then her husband noticed that, from time to time, Darlene was extremely cheerful. She talked very fast, switching from one topic to another, and seemed to have endless energy, yet she slept only one or two hours a night: "I don't know what happens to her sometimes. It's like she's on speed—she just goes on and on and *on*." Her husband also noticed that she was acting in ways she had never done before the accident. She was quick to anger and cursed often. Darlene also started spending lavishly on things she had and did not need—expensive perfumes, clothes, shoes, handbags, and high-end jewelry. These periods would last for about a week to ten days, and then her mood slowly returned to normal. She wasn't irritable or agitated, and she rarely got upset over anything—she was back to the "old" Darlene.

Two years after the accident, however, during yet another episode, Darlene became so angry that she tried to jump out of the attic window. Her husband stopped her just in time and called her doctor, who admitted Darlene to an acute-care psychiatric facility. Her husband told the admitting staff that Darlene had experienced three such episodes over the two years since the accident. These episodes were similar to some of the episodes her brother had experienced, he told them, but he insisted that Darlene had never exhibited these symptoms before her TBI.

Darlene stayed in the hospital for about two weeks and was treated with both an antipsychotic, Seroquel (quetiapine), and a mood stabilizer, Depakote (valproic acid). She responded very well to the combined medications and was discharged to an outpatient facility with recommendations for regular follow-up.

ONE OF THE EMOTIONAL DISORDERS that can occur after traumatic brain injury is mania. Mania is a state of heightened mental and physical activity. Everything about the person with mania is speeded up—elated mood, excess energy, racing thoughts, and almost frantic activity.

Some people hearing about mania wonder why it is considered a problem. After all, most of us probably wouldn't mind some extra energy, and the feeling of euphoria seems desirable. Unfortunately, along with the increased energy and euphoria, other symptoms of mania, such as impulsivity and reckless behaviors, can cause problems.

Symptoms

Classic symptoms of mania are a decreased need for sleep (for days), racing thoughts, grandiose thoughts, rapid-fire speech that is hard to interrupt, exaggerated or irritable mood, restlessness, and impulsivity. It's common for people in a manic state to go for days without sleeping or to sleep only for a few hours a night. They initiate many tasks at once yet fail to complete any of them, and they can exhibit abnormal goal-directed behavior, such as spending sprees or an overactive sex drive. Aggression, edginess, hallucinations, and delusions are also common in mania. These symptoms may get out of control, interfere with day-to-day activities, and require hospitalization.

In the person with TBI, these manifestations of mania may be intermittent and episodic, but some symptoms, such as irritability, mild aggression, and impulsivity, may persist and become part of the person's new baseline personality. The medical diagnosis in such cases is "personality change secondary to traumatic brain injury." When treating a person with these symptoms, clinicians may call family members to find out if the heightened state of activity is persistent or intermittent.

Darlene, because she had normal mood states between her episodes, with no irritability, agitation, or aggression, was suffering only from mania, not a permanent personality change. The person with TBI should be evaluated as soon as possible for these aggressive behaviors because hyperexcitability and impulsivity can lead to reckless and dangerous behavior; remember, Darlene tried to jump out the window.

In a person who has had a traumatic brain injury, mania, or a milder version called hypomania, can combine with personality changes due to the brain injury. Mania is time limited—lasting days to weeks—but personality change secondary to TBI is more persistent and may be permanent.

Mania can occur as part of bipolar (or manic-depressive) illness not related to brain injury. We believe bipolar disorder is predominantly a genetically based illness. In bipolar disorder, a manic phase alternates with depression. Mania that develops after a TBI can look the same as the mania of bipolar disorder.

Research suggests that mania after TBI often develops in people with injuries to the frontal and temporal lobes. We know that brain shrinkage and damage to the prefrontal cortex, amygdala, and basal ganglia can also cause mania. Unbalanced levels of the brain chemicals serotonin, dopamine, and norepinephrine may also be related to bipolar disorder. Some researchers suggest a "double-hit" theory: that is, manic episodes occur after brain injury in those who already have some predisposing factors, such as a family history of bipolar disorder.

Treatment

Acute worsening of mood or sudden change in mood state in a person with TBI needs immediate medical evaluation. In many cases, the person with TBI may not recognize that her symptoms are worsening. Family members should contact the person's doctor immediately; if the doctor cannot be reached, the family should take the person to be evaluated in the closest emergency department. Acute exacerbation requires immediate treatment with medications; mood stabilizers and antipsychotics are typical treatments for mania. Common mood stabilizers are lithium, Depakote (valproic acid), and Tegretol (carbamazepine). Seroquel (quetiapine), Risperdal (risperidone), and Zyprexa (olanzapine) are examples of antipsychotics.

After mood stabilization, it is important for the person to continue outpatient treatment, as Darlene did. Outpatient treatment focuses on monitoring signs and symptoms, observing medication compliance, and adjusting medications as needed. Some of these medications require the patient to have regular blood work done, to check the drug levels in the blood. Low doses may not be effective, and high doses can be toxic.

It is best for the person with TBI-induced mania to abstain from using alcohol and illicit drugs. Mood-altering substances can make the symptoms of mania worse, particularly impulsivity, and impulsivity prompts risky behaviors.

Behavioral and talk therapy can be helpful in combination with medication. These therapies include supportive therapy, focusing on education about TBI and mood symptoms (in both the early and later stages of the diagnosis), and healthy strategies to prevent or minimize stress, since stress can be a trigger for a manic episode.

In summary, untreated mania is a potentially dangerous condition because people with mania have minimal insight into their illness and may indulge in risky and life-threatening behaviors. As a family member or caregiver, helping the person with TBI experiencing mania seek professional treatment and ensuring they remain compliant will go a long way toward preventing or at least minimizing manic episodes. Stressors can worsen episodes of mania, so reduce stress as much as possible and work with your loved one to help her handle stress. If you notice early signs of relapse—sleeping less than usual, becoming more irritable or euphoric for no particular reason, or excessive energy and activity—encourage her to see her doctor.

Tips for Coping with Mania

If you are experiencing mania after TBI:

> ❯ Do not adjust or stop medications without first consulting your doctor. Compliance with treatment even after resolving the manic crisis is important for continued improvement after TBI.
> ❯ Avoid using alcohol and illicit drugs. Continued use of alcohol and other mind-altering drugs can worsen mood states, which is why people with TBI or mania after TBI need to abstain from their use. If you find that you cannot stop using alcohol or drugs on your own, seek professional help.

If you know someone who is experiencing mania after TBI:

> ❯ Consult with the doctor early. Seek medical help as soon as possible if you notice a sudden change in mood and behavior, to establish the diagnosis and get treatment.
> ❯ Be careful and gentle, yet firm. The person who is going through a manic phase may have limited or no awareness of her problem and may refuse treatment.
> ❯ Call 911 if you are concerned about safety. Safety comes first and trumps all other issues. Someone in a manic episode may be agitated or even aggressive. If there are concerns about safety, and she is unwilling to go to the hospital, call 911 or get immediate help.
> ❯ Encourage your loved one to maintain a healthy lifestyle. Shift work and changes in sleep patterns can precipitate manic episodes. Work with her to maintain a strict sleep schedule, keep good sleep habits (see "Sleep Hygiene" in Chapter 12), get regular exercise, and eat a balanced diet.

Ask whether she can change work schedules to avoid early-morning or late-night shift work. Staying awake longer and longer at night might be a clue that the person with brain injury is beginning a manic episode.

> Minimize or manage stress. Be aware that excessive or unmanaged stress can trigger a manic episode. Learn what triggers manic episodes (such as noncompliance with medications or alcohol use) in the person you are caring for and help her to reduce or avoid these stressors.

> Learn about mania, medications, and signs of early relapse. Being knowledgeable about TBI and mood disturbances can be very useful in preventing or reducing the frequency of relapses.

8

Apathy

Tony was carrying a box of holiday decorations down from his attic when he missed a step, tumbled down the stairs, and cracked his head on the tile floor. He sustained a severe TBI, and emergency department doctors worked fast to remove blood from the right front side of his brain. Tony had a long recovery, including a stay at a rehabilitation hospital followed by intensive physical and speech therapies. But when he returned home, Tony seemed to slow down. He appeared disengaged and uninterested in everyday activities. His wife worried, concerned that this attitude could not be healthy for Tony's brain recovery. She wondered how much of this behavior was just his being lazy and how much was due to the brain injury: "He's just a couch potato these days. He doesn't do anything!"

After much prodding from his wife, Tony agreed to see his primary care doctor. When his doctor questioned him about his mood state, Tony replied that he wasn't actually sad, he just felt "dull." His wife added that Tony was eating and sleeping well, and he wasn't feeling hopeless or as if he was a burden to her. Tony's primary care doctor referred him to a psychiatrist with expertise in brain injury. After detailed evaluation, the neuropsychiatrist determined that 54-year-old Tony was suffering from a lack of motivation and diagnosed him with post-TBI apathy syndrome.

MOVING ON FROM CHAPTER 7'S discussion of a state of heightened energy and motivation (mania), we discuss in this chapter a state quite the opposite—that of decreased motivation. Motivation is a murky concept, but we all intuitively have a sense of what it is. We can think of motivation as the ability to set a goal and take steps to achieve that goal. Typically, the things we are interested in are the things that motivate us. Other motivators might be the need to feed our families, pride in our work, or religious or ideological beliefs. Motivation is what gets us up in the morning, spurs us to do the many things we do in a typical day, and pushes us to persevere despite the inevitable setbacks in our days and our lives.

Apathy is a decrease in or lack of motivation, and it develops in many people who have neurological problems such as dementia, stroke, and Parkinson's disease. It can occur alone or in combination with major depression or schizophrenia.

Apathy is common in traumatic brain injury. Post-TBI apathy is associated with less recovery and less response to treatment. This outcome is not surprising, given that a person with TBI who is not an active participant in physical therapy or speech therapy is likely to make only limited progress.

Often, apathy results from direct trauma to circuits in subcortical areas deep within the brain, including the thalamus, amygdala, and basal ganglia. A part of the basal ganglia called the ventral striatum is particularly important in our ability to sense pleasure and be motivated to act so that we achieve pleasure. Interactions between these areas and the prefrontal cortex (especially the dorsolateral prefrontal cortex) and the anterior cingulate lead to motivation. Damage to these areas and circuits can lead to apathy. The frontal lobes, unfortunately, are particularly vulnerable to brain trauma. Furthermore, TBI often stretches or otherwise damages the axon tracts connecting these subcortical structures to the frontal lobe, and this damage leads to disruption of the motivation circuitry.

Symptoms

The person with TBI does not typically complain of feeling apathy. Rather, caregivers or family members notice the personality change. Perhaps they see that the person with TBI doesn't finish tasks during rehabilitation or at home or that he isn't following through with things he has committed to. Perhaps he makes plans for the next day but doesn't follow through, so plans never come to fruition. The person with TBI may not commit to any goals at all. People with apathy often seem to be perfectly content just "being" and not particularly interested in "doing." Family members may complain that their loved one is "being lazy" or is a "couch potato" or that he doesn't "sparkle" any more. They may think his personality has changed—he is no longer the vivacious, fun-loving, interested person they have known for so long. Now, he's pleasant enough, but flat.

Apathy after TBI is a common cause of conflict between the person with TBI experiencing apathy and his family or caregivers. The family may feel that their loved one is not putting forth full effort and may become frustrated with him. They may feel that they are putting in hard work on his behalf, while he has become lazy and is doing very little. They may feel that he will waste the significant expense of rehabilitation therapy.

Apathy is often a direct consequence of the injury, but it can also be due to other medical problems. Thyroid problems, infection, anemia, low testosterone, Parkinson's disease, Alzheimer's disease, vitamin deficiency, sleep problems, and environmental factors, among others, can all cause symptoms of apathy. Blood tests can rule out thyroid problems, vitamin deficiencies, anemia, and infection, so ask the doctor whether blood testing would be appropriate.

Consider not only general medical causes but also illicit drug use and medications as causes of apathy. Marijuana, alcohol, and narcotic pain medications are associated with apathy. Even selective serotonin reuptake inhibitors and similar agents used to treat depression and anxiety can, in some people, cause apathy.

It is sometimes difficult to distinguish between apathy and depression. Tony, in our opening story, for example, had symptoms predominantly of apathy, not symptoms of depression, such as sadness, feelings of hopelessness or guilt, or changes in sleep or appetite.

Of course, it is possible for a person with TBI to have both apathy and depression. Apathy can be part of depression, but it is not always present in people who have depression. Conversely, depression can, but does not always, occur along with apathy. One way to distinguish between the two is to note that the core issues with major depression are lack of enjoyment and persistent low mood. The depressed person typically has poor self-esteem and little self-regard. The depressed person may also report feelings of hopelessness or suicidal thoughts or both. In contrast, the person with apathy may not feel or appear particularly sad. A person with apathy may deny that he can't enjoy things; he is simply not interested in initiating or engaging in activities that could lead to enjoyment. In fact, he may be quite content doing nothing.

Diagnosis

It is important to distinguish apathy from depression, not only to make an accurate diagnosis, but also because treatment can be different. As noted above, some antidepressants can actually make people apathetic, so it's best to avoid certain antidepressants if the issue is truly one of apathy. On the other hand, some antidepressants do help apathy, so talk with the doctor to determine which antidepressant—if any—is best for the person with apathy. Some antidepressants are helpful for people who may have both apathy and depression.

To more accurately diagnose apathy, the doctor may use a formal rating scale such as the Apathy Evaluation Scale. Typically, the doctor asks the caregiver pointed questions about how the person with TBI is doing. Be as open and honest as you can in answering these questions because your responses will help the doctor make an accurate diagnosis.

Treatment

Scientists believe that, at a neurochemical level, dopamine is an important contributor to motivation. The release of dopamine associated with something in our environment appears to make that stimulus more relevant, or salient, to us. In other words, dopamine allows the brain to tell itself, so to speak, that something out there is important. Dopamine prods our brains to engage in action.

Perhaps not coincidentally, dopamine is involved in the control of movements. Increasing dopamine can thus increase motivation. Scientists believe that dopamine is critical for the "want" system of the brain, the circuit of the brain that drives our wants, housed primarily in the ventral striatum in the basal ganglia. Medications that are predominantly stimulating and increase dopamine are used in the treatment of apathy.

Environmental and Behavioral Therapies and Lifestyle Changes

Behavioral and environmental methods are very important in the treatment of apathy. We recommend trying environmental and behavioral methods first prior to using medications because they have no side effects. If other possible causes of apathy (narcotic pain medications; high doses of SSRIs; alcohol, marijuana, or illicit drugs; medical disorders) are eliminated or addressed and apathy does not resolve, then a helpful approach may be to have the person with TBI work with a professional, such as an occupational therapist (OT), to learn how to structure his days. Examples include mapping out a timetable for every day of the week that includes set times to do routine activities (bathing or taking meals, for example), enjoyable activities, exercise, and rest, establishing sleep time and wake time, and making to-do lists based on priorities. It is also helpful to build in rewards that the person can earn for following the timetable or completing tasks. Verbal cues (that is, telling your loved one what to do and patiently reminding him) may be helpful. Problem-solving training by an occupational therapist or a psychotherapist may also be helpful. Music therapy and singing can help. Having more stimulation in the environment can be activating as well. A treatment known as Snoezelen multisensory environmental therapy may reduce apathy, but research in this area is scant.

Drug Therapy

Medications that increase dopamine include bromocriptine and stimulants such as Ritalin (methylphenidate) and Adderall (dextroamphetamine). These medications are used to treat apathy and seem to help some people, but they have not been adequately studied to determine that they are indeed beneficial. Amantadine, which indirectly affects dopamine, can successfully treat apathy, but it too has not been adequately studied. Some doctors prescribe certain antidepressants to treat apathy, including Effexor (venlafaxine), Pristiq (desvenlafaxine), and Wellbutrin (bupropion). Other agents to consider include Sinemet (carbidopa-levodopa) and Eldepryl (selegiline). Finally, a class of medications called acetylcholinesterase inhibitors (which increase acetylcholine), which includes medications like Aricept (donepezil), Exelon (rivastigmine), and Razadyne (galantamine), can help with apathy in dementia and so may be helpful in TBI as well. All of these medications, however, can have serious side effects, such as changes in heart rate or blood pressure, confusion, or delirium if taken in inappropriate dosage and without regular supervision by a physician.

In summary, apathy is not uncommon after TBI. Apathy is lack of motivation that can affect a person emotionally (making him feel dull, for example), behaviorally (causing trouble initiating and keeping up with tasks), and cognitively (slowing the processing of information). Apathy can occur with or without depression. Apathy after TBI can be a major contributor to poor recovery. Family and caregivers must recognize apathy as a symptom of traumatic brain injury and be aware that the person with TBI may be apathetic as a direct or an indirect result of the brain injury. People who were not apathetic before their injury are unlikely to become less active just because they are being lazy or resistant. Once you know that, you can help the person with apathy receive appropriate treatment and help him through his recovery.

Tips for Coping with Apathy after TBI
If you know someone who is experiencing apathy after TBI:

> Educate yourself about apathy. Apathy is not laziness. It is a condition in which a person's internal motivating system is not working well. Do not blame the person with TBI who is apathetic.

> Get involved. Use external motivators to motivate the person with apathy. As a caregiver, you can get him involved in hobbies or other pleasurable activities. Start by encouraging him to do things that you know he enjoyed before the brain injury. Gradually introduce other activities and responsibilities, such as completing certain tasks (taking out the trash, getting the mail, for example) or participating in group efforts (decorating a holiday tree with the family, for example).

> If appropriate for the person with TBI, request a referral to an occupational therapist who can work with him to plan and structure his days.

> Certain drugs and medications (marijuana, narcotics, or tranquilizers) can cause or worsen apathy and are best avoided. If you think that any medication your loved one is taking may be causing or worsening the apathy, discuss your concerns with his doctor.

PART III

Behavioral Problems Caused by the Traumatized Brain

In this part of the book, we explore behavioral problems that often occur after TBI. These behavioral problems can include psychosis, aggression, impulsivity, and sleep disturbances. Behavioral problems, as you might imagine, can be a serious concern for family members of a person who has sustained a traumatic brain injury. Not only can the behavioral problems cause problems within the family, but they may affect recovery from the brain injury. While physical injuries are obvious, behavioral problems may be hidden in some ways. Behavioral consequences from the TBI may be unexpected, or there may be a failure to recognize or make the connection between the behavior and the TBI. Such misunderstandings can make behavioral problems after traumatic brain injury especially troubling.

9

Psychosis

Lisa worked hard and saved for her dream vacation—a ski trip to the Colorado mountains with three close friends to celebrate her 27th birthday. On their last day on the mountain slope, Lisa collided with another skier and slammed the side of her head into a pine tree. She was airlifted to the emergency department and diagnosed with severe traumatic brain injury. Once she was stable, Lisa was transported to her hometown hospital, where she remained for several weeks, and then she continued with extensive rehabilitation. Not long after she returned home to her parents and younger brother she developed seizures, for which her doctor prescribed an antiseizure medication.

About a year after the accident, Lisa began having suspicious thoughts that an old high school teacher was going to kill her and her family. She became convinced that she had to perform several rituals to keep the teacher away from her loved ones. Among the actions she felt compelled to do were to spin around three times in a clockwise direction followed by spinning around five times in a counterclockwise direction and to arrange magazines in a certain way on the dining room table. Her family was puzzled at first and then grew frustrated by her compulsion to perform these rituals. Her mother explained to Lisa's doctor that Lisa had had no contact or communication with the teacher for many years.

TRAUMATIC BRAIN INJURY CAN TRIGGER the onset of psychosis. The words *psychosis* and *psychotic symptoms* refer to delusions, hallucinations, or illogical thinking. In other words, psychosis is a state in which the sufferer is not in touch with reality. In this chapter, we discuss the various forms psychotic symptoms can take after TBI.

Symptoms

Delusions are fixed false beliefs that a person holds despite evidence to the contrary. For example, Lisa in our opening story had delusions that her old teacher was going to kill her and her family. Lisa firmly believed this, even though she had not heard from the teacher for years and despite repeated assurances from her family that there was no threat. She also held the firm belief that, by doing certain things, she could prevent the teacher from harming her or her family.

Paranoid delusions, in particular, are typical of post-TBI psychosis. Just as in Lisa's case, people with paranoid delusions have the unshakeable belief that someone is watching them or targeting them, even if there is evidence to the contrary. People who have paranoid delusions are convinced that their lives are in danger, that they must always be vigilant, and that they are at risk of significant bodily harm. Cognitive deficits can add to such paranoia. For example, if a paranoid person can't remember where she placed certain things (keys, purse), her paranoia can escalate into believing that someone is entering her house and stealing these items from her.

Psychosis can also include hallucinations. A person who hallucinates sees, hears, smells, or feels things that are not really there, but those hallucinations are as real as anything else in her experience. These perceptions can be frightening and can lead to agitation and anxiety. A person with TBI may have auditory hallucinations consisting of conversations between two people about her. Such hallucinations may consist of hearing people arguing about her, or mumbling in a way that she cannot fully understand. If she overhears an imagined "conversation" coming from another room, she may go to investigate and discover no one there. She may hear inanimate objects such as a lamp, a desk, or even the carpet speaking to her.

Illogical thinking, in which thoughts are jumbled or disorganized, is another form of psychosis. The person with TBI who experiences this usually does not complain about these symptoms for the simple reason that she is not aware that there's a problem. Family members usually take the person to a doctor when they notice her strange behavior. The illogical thinking may be so severe that others cannot understand what she is saying.

Other symptoms of psychosis include odd behavior such as holding a two-way conversation with oneself, laughing or grinning inappropriately, or a sudden behavioral change—withdrawing socially or ignoring personal hygiene, for example.

Risk Factors

Psychotic symptoms are more common in people who have had TBIs, particularly those with severe TBIs, compared with those who have not. Psychosis may be more likely after TBI if the brain was vulnerable because of preexisting brain damage associated with a birth or learning disability, even if relatively mild. Other factors that increase the risk of psychosis after traumatic brain injury are traumatic brain injury in early childhood and a personal or family history of psychosis or schizophrenia.

The strongest of these risk factors is the severity of the TBI; that is, people with severe TBI are far more likely to have psychosis than those with mild TBI. And the more severe the TBI, the greater the likelihood of having seizures, and having seizures further increases the risk of psychotic symptoms.

Some people who develop psychotic symptoms after TBI have a family history of a psychotic disorder like schizophrenia or had milder psychotic symptoms before the brain injury. Similarly, having a TBI elevates the risk for developing schizophrenia in those who have a family history of schizophrenia, particularly if that person is a first-degree relative (parent, child, or sibling) of the person with schizophrenia.

Some people with TBI psychosis may not develop the full spectrum of schizophrenia symptoms (such as hallucinations and delusions) but develop only what are called negative symptoms. Some examples of negative symptoms are lack of motivation, poor thinking skills, lack of speech, and lack of emotion. Other people with TBI do not develop these negative symptoms but experience only delusions, such as believing that family members are not who they are, but are imposters, or that a particular place has been duplicated and is present in two different sites.

The timing of post-TBI psychosis varies. Sometimes psychosis develops immediately after the brain injury and often in the context of delirium. People experiencing delirium become confused as to where they are and what is happening to them. They may have frightening visual hallucinations: they may see armies marching into their hospital room threatening to shoot them or fantastical animals flying in the room, perhaps chimeras, who transform themselves into monsters with gnashing teeth. They may see hospital staff stealthily mixing poison into their intravenous fluids. They may see their caregivers transforming into demons, ready to eviscerate them. Such hallucinations can be terrifying, even overwhelming, for the person with TBI.

Psychotic symptoms in the context of delirium can stem from multiple factors. In some cases, the brain injury itself is the direct cause. Alternatively, certain medications, lack of oxygen, and several concurrent medical problems like blood loss or anemia can also cause delirium. Scientists believe that delirium develops in response to a decrease in a brain chemical called acetylcholine. This chemical is also important for dreaming. If we consider delirium as a dream state, in which dreams mix with consciousness, it may be a state of consciousness between wakefulness and dreaming. Psychotic symptoms can also develop months or years after a TBI. It is not clear why this happens, although it seems that people who have injuries to the temporal lobe may be more prone to this later onset. It may be that as the brain reorganizes after the injury, faulty "rewiring" allows psychotic symptoms to occur. There is evidence, in fact, that dysfunction of the white matter (the axon tracts that connect different parts of the brain) is related to psychotic symptoms. Injury to these tracts could lead to poor crosstalk between sections of the brain and eventually to psychosis.

Damage to the frontal lobes, basal ganglia, and hippocampi is also associated with psychosis (see figures 2.1a and b). The hippocampi are seahorse-shaped structures deep within the brain inside the temporal lobes. The hippocampi are important in retaining short-term memory. It is also clear, however, that the hippocampi are smaller than normal in people who have schizophrenia, and damage to the hippocampus may be related to psychosis.

Lisa in our opening story had severe TBI, seizures associated with TBI, and psychosis in the form of persecution-type delusions that developed several months after the TBI. Lisa's case is a typical presentation of TBI psychosis.

Treatment

People with TBI who experience hallucinations or delusions should undergo a thorough evaluation, including a magnetic resonance imaging (MRI) of the brain and possibly an electroencephalogram (EEG), a recording of the electrical activity in the brain. The doctor should make note of what medications the patient is taking, to rule out either medications or concurrent medical problems as the source of the delirium. The doctor will take steps to rule out substance use disorder because certain drugs of abuse can cause or worsen psychotic symptoms. Cocaine, amphetamines, methamphetamines, LSD, Ecstasy, "bath salts," and marijuana, among others, can cause psychotic symptoms.

If the person with TBI exhibits psychotic symptoms, she is not being purposefully difficult. She is likely agitated because her hallucinations are frightening to her. She may believe that her caregiver or family is trying to harm her and so may lash out and resist any efforts to help.

Antipsychotic medications are commonly prescribed to treat psychosis. Examples include Risperdal (risperidone), Haldol (haloperidol), Zyprexa (olanzapine), Seroquel (quetiapine), Abilify (aripiprazole), Latuda (lurasidone), and Clozaril (clozapine). Antipsychotic medications work by lowering the amount of a neurotransmitter in the brain called dopamine. A simplistic explanation is that excess dopamine in one particular tract of the brain is associated with the production of psychotic symptoms. Antipsychotics can help with psychotic symptoms by reducing dopamine.

Unfortunately, persons with psychotic symptoms often have poor insight into their condition. In other words, they may not think there is anything wrong with them, or they may believe that they can deal with the situation on their own. In either case, they may not want to take their medication. If you are a caregiver, emphasize to your loved one just how important it is that she take the antipsychotic medication, at least for the short term. People with TBI psychosis may have psychotic symptoms for the short term and may not have to be on antipsychotic medications permanently.

Arguing with a person with TBI psychosis about her beliefs is unproductive and can, in fact, lead to agitation. Delusions are by definition fixed, and it is unlikely that you will be successful in convincing the person with TBI psychosis that her beliefs are false. The same is true for hallucinations; after all, to the person who sees or hears them, those hallucinations are real.

As family, friend, or caregiver, you can best serve the person with TBI by being understanding and supportive and by encouraging her to take her medications and to follow her doctor's advice.

It can be disheartening to see your family member in the hospital because of psychosis. She may beg and plead for you to get her out. Understand that she is in the emergency department or in the hospital for good reason. Today, most hospital stays are short, a few days to a week or two. To prevent rehospitalization, it is crucial to encourage and make sure the person you are caring for takes her medication(s).

In summary, psychosis after TBI can occur, but it is less likely to develop than depression or anxiety. Psychotic symptoms may develop after the injury as part of an acute confusional state or they may develop months to years later. Luckily, medications are available to reduce these symptoms quite effectively. Dealing with someone who has psychotic symptoms can be distressing, but it may be reassuring to hear that many people do get better with the appropriate treatment. Understanding that people with TBI psychosis are exhibiting bewildering or odd behaviors because of the damage to their brain can help you, as a caregiver, empathize and be supportive to the person you are caring for.

Tips for Coping with Psychosis after TBI

If you know someone who is experiencing psychosis after TBI:

> Educate yourself about psychosis. Learn about the symptoms, medications, triggers for relapse, and people or physicians to call in case of an emergency.

> If you are concerned about the safety of your loved one, take her to the nearest hospital or call 911. If she is agitated, do not try to restrain her. If she is unwilling to go to the hospital, you must call 911. A person having a psychotic episode may feel threatened and react aggressively in self-defense. A person in the midst of a psychotic episode can be very strong, perhaps because she believes she is fighting for her life. She may not appreciate that someone is trying to help her. Instead, she may think you or others are part of the conspiracy against her or that you are not who you say you are. If your loved one becomes agitated and aggressive, it is best to call 911.

> If your loved one is describing abnormal experiences, respond to her feelings, not her words. She may be frightened. Show your support—respect the person and her abnormal beliefs even when you know they are not true. You may feel you are tricking your loved one or lying by not correcting her thinking. It is more productive to reframe this. The goal is not to make your loved one understand the truth, for the psychotic process eliminates her ability to appreciate the truth. The goal is to make her feel safe and less distressed. If possible, help her to calm down, talk to her or engage her in something enjoyable. Such redirection of focus may distract her from her tormenting thoughts or stimuli. Replacing negative thoughts and experiences with something positive may calm her.

> Never argue with a person with TBI psychosis. Trying to convince your loved one that it is all in her mind or calling her crazy is counterproductive and in fact may make her more agitated and even aggressive.
> When the person is upset or agitated about the psychotic symptoms, give her space. Speak calmly, in short sentences, and when necessary, give firm and clear directions. Keep in mind that she may be distracted by voices or unusual thoughts, so give only one direction at a time.

10

Aggression

As Lee walked through a store parking lot headed for his car, another car backed out from a parking space and knocked him down. Lee's head hit the pavement and he lost consciousness. An ambulance took him to the nearest emergency department, where a brain scan showed bleeding in the space between his skull and brain. Brain surgeons immediately removed the blood clot. The operation was successful—Lee was healthy and strong at 23—but he had a prolonged hospital stay and required extensive rehabilitation. While in the hospital, Lee developed seizures and had episodes of agitation immediately after he was admitted, but both conditions resolved over time.

After Lee returned home, he had emotional outbursts over trivial matters. For example, a minor disagreement at the dinner table with his family escalated into a shouting match, and Lee stormed off, punching holes in walls. At one point, Lee became so enraged over an empty cereal box that he wrenched the cupboard door off its hinges. Lee's wife reported, "The children are terrified of him now." Because of these aggressive episodes, it has been hard for Lee to get into a day program whose goal is to help him transition back to work.

AGGRESSION IS HOSTILE, harmful, or destructive behavior that can be physical or verbal and can range from irritability to physical assault on others. Aggression can manifest as cursing, threatening, hitting, pushing, yelling, or breaking or throwing things. Physical aggression, in particular, can be disturbing to caregivers and disruptive to recovery for the person with TBI. An outburst of aggression from a previously calm person may be scary for caregivers to deal with. Aggression may also frighten the person with TBI himself; he may feel out of control, not like his normal self. People who develop aggression after TBI may need to be medicated, perhaps even placed in a medical facility for monitoring. For you, as a caregiver, to provide the best support for your loved one, you must understand how aggression can occur after TBI and how best to manage it, for your own safety and the safety of others.

Aggression is, unfortunately, common after TBI. It is more common after repeated injuries and severe injuries. Risk factors for developing aggression after TBI include being male, having a TBI at a young age, alcohol or substance abuse problems before the TBI, injury to specific parts of the brain affected by the TBI, and the onset of mood problems after the TBI. Alcohol or substance abuse after TBI can release inhibitions, making the person with TBI more vulnerable to acting out aggressively.

Symptoms

Certain patterns and features tend to occur with aggressive behavior after TBI. The aggression typically is reactive, that is, triggered by a specific thing or event, even a very minor stress. In Lee's case, in our opening story, trivial disagreements made him agitated and aggressive. The aggressive reaction can be entirely disproportionate to the issue at hand.

Aggressive behaviors after TBI tend to be impulsive, without planning or forethought. Typically, the person with TBI doesn't mull over a perceived slight, start getting angry, and then plan what to say or do. Rather, the response to a trigger is sudden and explosive, without gradual buildup. Aggression after TBI is thus not criminal violence, in which criminals plot and plan, execute a crime, then make their planned escape.

Just as aggression after TBI typically builds up suddenly, it also dies down abruptly; it is not usually a sustained state lasting days or weeks. Indeed, people with TBI usually regret their outburst. They tend to be embarrassed and upset by their own behavior. They tend not to blame others and do not justify their behavior.

Aggression can occur soon after TBI or months later. Aggression soon after the TBI, in the context of confusion and disorientation, is most likely due to delirium. This aggressive behavior is the direct result of the trauma to the brain and the subsequent alterations in body physiology or of medications administered after the TBI, such as pain medications. In the context of delirium, the person's thinking is muddled; he may be confused about where he is or what happened. This uncertainty may fluctuate; he may seem "with it" at times and completely confused at other times. When he is confused, he may act out aggressively to defend himself. He may believe he is in the middle of a war zone, or in a fantastical world of demons. He may have visual hallucinations, perhaps seeing frightening displays of aggression by his imagined monsters.

In a hospital setting, aggression due to delirium is usually treated with medication. Doctors use these medications temporarily while the brain recovers from the immediate shock of the trauma. The TBI can also cause other medical problems, which can also cause delirium. Infections can develop, sodium or calcium or magnesium levels can be abnormal, or blood oxygen levels can fall. Treating and resolving these issues can help manage the delirium, but doctors often use antipsychotic medications as well. If required, antipsychotics are necessary for a limited time, but they are necessary not only to reduce the aggression and make sure no one (including the person with TBI) is harmed but also because they may reduce the duration of the delirium.

Medications can also lead to delirium, and the doctor will evaluate any medications the person with TBI is taking. Certain medicines that reduce a neurotransmitter called acetylcholine are particularly important to investigate because they can cause delirium. These include medicines like Benadryl (diphenhydramine) or bladder medications like Ditropan (oxybutynin), among many others. If the person with TBI was drinking large quantities of alcohol before the TBI, he may be in alcohol withdrawal, which can certainly cause aggression. People who were regularly taking benzodiazepines, for example, Ativan (lorazepam), Xanax (alprazolam), or Klonopin (clonazepam), before the injury may also experience withdrawal. A person going through withdrawal from alcohol or benzodiazepines may be restless, sweaty, shaky, and sensitive to light or sound, have a rapid heartbeat or high blood pressure, or have hallucinations. Withdrawal from pain medicines (opiates like Vicodin [hydrocodone/acetaminophen], OxyContin [oxycodone], or Percocet [oxycodone/acetaminophen]) can also cause agitation and aggression. Drugs like cocaine, amphetamines, or PCP can cause aggression as well.

After a TBI (particularly a severe TBI), seizures can occur, and seizures may be associated or followed by aggression. In general, if related to seizures, the aggression is brief and not directed towards anyone. Other causes of aggression soon after a TBI include metabolic disturbances such as low blood sugar or change in blood sodium levels. The doctors will investigate all these possibilities as causes for the aggression. Sometimes it is not just one thing but a combination of things that leads to delirium and aggression.

After the immediate post-TBI period, the person with TBI may develop aggression for many other reasons. He might be susceptible to other medical problems; for example, he may be vulnerable to falls, and if he hits his head again, he could bleed into the brain or develop seizures. He could develop significant depression, and manifest his internal, psychic pain physically. He may develop severe anxiety and lash out at people or things because he has trouble expressing his anger. He may have nightmares or recurrent thoughts of the incident that led to the TBI (combat or a car accident, for example), and develop posttraumatic stress disorder. Pain that follows a TBI can also cause agitation and aggression. Trouble adjusting to a new level of functioning, becoming dependent on family or friends, or feeling sorry for himself and bitter about what fate has dealt him—all these swirling emotions can lead to aggression in the person with TBI. Finally, the TBI itself can affect parts of the brain that control emotions, including anger, and lead to long-term problems with aggression.

Damage to specific areas of the brain leads to aggression (see figures 2.1a and b). The frontal lobes and temporal lobes are prone to injury in TBI, and these are the very areas critical to controlling our impulses to anger. Damage to the lower part of the frontal lobes (the orbitofrontal part of the prefrontal cortex) and the front of the

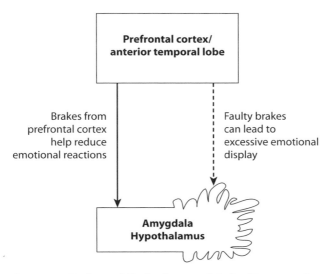

Figure 10.1. Regions of the brain associated with aggression

temporal lobes (the anterior temporal lobes) is most closely associated with aggression. The amygdala, deep within the emotional brain (or limbic system), is also important for aggression and is involved in emotional regulation. Activation of the amygdala can spark outrage or an exaggerated response to perceived slights—exactly the form of aggression often seen in TBI. Finally, the hypothalamus may play a role in aggression because it is responsible for fight-or-flight reactions; stimulation of areas in the hypothalamus can lead to aggressive behavior.

There might be a circuit involving the orbitofrontal cortex, anterior temporal lobe, amygdala, and hypothalamus that is critical in controlling our aggressive impulses (figure 10.1). The aggressive impulses generated by the amygdala and the hypothalamus are probably normally regulated by the orbitofrontal cortex and perhaps the anterior temporal lobe. In other words, these cortical areas of the brain may act as a "brake" on the aggressive impulses of the emotional brain. Damage to these frontal or temporal areas deactivates the "brake," as it were, setting loose the emotional brain's aggressive impulses.

On another level, we can look at the neurotransmitters that are associated with aggression. Norepinephrine, dopamine, serotonin, acetylcholine, and GABA may all play roles in aggressive behavior. Increased norepinephrine or dopamine, or decreased serotonin or GABA, can be associated with aggression. Increased acetylcholine may also be associated with aggression, although this correlation is less clear than with the other neurotransmitters just mentioned.

There might also be a genetic predisposition to aggression after TBI expressed by a gene for an enzyme called monoamine oxidase type A (MAO-A). This enzyme is important in breaking down dopamine, norepinephrine, and serotonin. People who have a genetic predilection for low levels of MAO-A may be more likely to be aggressive when provoked, presumably because they cannot break down some of these neurotransmitters (particularly norepinephrine and dopamine) effectively.

Treatment

The best treatment for aggression depends on whether the aggression is acute or chronic. Acute aggression lasts up to a few weeks, whereas chronic aggression extends beyond that.

Environmental and Behavioral Therapies and Lifestyle Changes

In treating chronic aggression after TBI, nonpharmacological approaches are an important part of treatment. Cognitive behavioral therapy (CBT) can help the person with TBI improve his coping skills, making it easier for him to manage his frustration. CBT also helps with depression and anxiety, both of which may be contributing to the aggression. Of course, the person with TBI must be at an injury level or recovery stage in which they have the cognitive abilities to benefit from CBT. CBT can also teach caregivers the coping skills they need to overcome their own frustrations as they try to help their loved ones.

For people who have severe traumatic brain injury, behavioral and environmental interventions are critical. These approaches involve assessing the antecedents to the behavior, the behavior itself, and the consequences of the behavior, also known as the ABCs of assessing behavior problems. Assessing the antecedents involves careful history taking and observations. Does it seem that the person with TBI is getting aggressive because he is not able to communicate properly? Does he get aggressive only with certain caregivers? If so, is it because those caregivers invade his personal space, for example? Could the physical environment or some discomfort be making him aggressive? Is his environment overstimulating him? Is he uncomfortable or in pain and has no way to express that other than aggression?

Assessing the aggressive behavior itself means observing the pattern in the behavior. Is the aggression verbal or physical? Does the person appear fearful? Could he be seeing hallucinations? Or is he lashing out only when someone touches him? Is it when he has nightmares? Is it when he doesn't sleep well?

The final step is to explore the consequences of the behavior. Sometimes caregivers may be inadvertently encouraging the aggression. For example, if the person with TBI doesn't get much attention except when he is aggressive, getting that attention, even if it is negative attention, may encourage the behavior further. If the aggression reflects hunger or pain or a need to use the toilet, simply reassuring or redirecting the person may increase aggression because the underlying issue hasn't been addressed.

Therapists who specialize in working with people who have brain injury are most qualified to perform these behavioral and environmental interventions, but caregivers should be aware of these principles as well. The professional may create a plan—in a rehabilitation setting, for example—and it is up to caregivers to implement the plan when the person with TBI returns home.

Drug Therapy

Aggression in the acute stage (which often stems from delirium) is treated with medications determined by the treating doctor. Benzodiazepines (lorazepam [Ativan], for example) may be used because they work quickly and are calming. However, it's best to avoid benzodiazepines except where alcohol or benzodiazepine withdrawal is responsible for the aggression; antipsychotics are an alternative.

There are medications for chronic aggression, and doctors often prescribe them in combination with the behavioral and environmental techniques discussed above. Beta blockers (which treat high blood pressure and cardiac issues), particularly Inderal (propranolol), are the most effective drugs for chronic aggression. Be aware, however, that it often takes weeks for these medications to take effect, and the doctor may need to adjust the dose several times to find the correct level for your loved one.

Antidepressants like Zoloft (sertraline), Celexa (citalopram), and Lexapro (escitalopram) may be helpful, not only for those with depression or anxiety along with the aggression, but also for their general effects on aggression. BuSpar (buspirone), an anti-anxiety agent, also seems to have anti-aggression effects in TBI.

Anticonvulsant medications can also be helpful, as they assist in stabilizing mood. Tegretol (carbamazepine) in particular seems to be beneficial. The doctor may also consider using Depakote (valproic acid). These medications help people with TBI who may have seizures associated with the injury, but they can also help with aggression even when there are no seizures.

Stimulants like Ritalin (methylphenidate) can be used, with caution, in certain cases. However, they can also worsen aggression in some people.

Finally, antipsychotic medications may be used in the long term for aggression as well, although they are best used when psychotic symptoms coincide with the aggression.

In summary, aggression after TBI can be disconcerting to all involved. Family and caregivers must recognize that aggression after TBI is often a consequence of factors beyond a person's control. As we have noted, there are multiple potential causes of the aggression, ranging from direct effects of the TBI, other medical issues, medications, and illicit drugs to adjustment and social factors. A number of pharmacological and nonpharmacological options are available to help control this behavior. Managing the aggression will allow the person with TBI to make a better recovery, stay at home, and return more quickly to a higher functioning level. With the help of physicians, therapists, and other specialists, you can help the person with TBI and aggression overcome this troubling behavior.

Tips for Coping with Aggression after TBI
If you know someone who is experiencing aggression after TBI:

> Call 911 if you are concerned about safety. Safety comes first, both the safety of the person experiencing aggression and that of those around him. If the aggression escalates and the person cannot calm down, call 911 or get immediate help.
> Respond, but don't react. When someone is having an aggressive outburst, reacting with anger or irritability only worsens the aggression. Do your best to respond to your loved one calmly and gently, speaking softly but clearly, while ensuring that the environment is safe.
> Be alert for aggression triggers and try to minimize or remove them. Triggers may be related to the environment (too much noise, bright lights, cluttered space, for example), people involved in your loved one's care (loud conversations, too many directions given at once), or something your loved one is doing or not doing (using alcohol or illicit drugs, sleeping poorly, taking certain medications). Learn what triggers aggression and take steps to avoid these triggers.
> Identify behavioral patterns of aggression. Channel the aggressive energy into healthier, safer activity. For example, if the person with aggression likes to throw things when he gets aggressive, give him a soft, squishy ball or a pillow and teach him to squeeze it when he feels angry. Teach him this behavior when he is calm and is willing to listen and learn. During an aggressive outburst, people are usually unable to learn any new techniques.
> Discuss the consequences of aggressive behavior with your loved one. Pick a time when he is calm to discuss his behavior and state specific consequences of such behavior: "If you ever threaten the children, I'll ask you to leave the house."

Be consistent with consequences, because inconsistent responses are confusing and can interfere with learning behavioral change.

> Think outside the box. Be creative; if the coping strategies you have devised just aren't working, keep searching for other methods to use. Seek guidance and help from doctors, therapists, or support groups.

11

Impulsivity

Kayla is 54 and an avid tennis player. While reaching to return a serve one morning, she stumbled, tripped, and fell sideways on the edge of the court, hitting her head on a concrete slab. The blow led to bleeding in the brain. The blood clot was surgically removed shortly after Kayla arrived in the emergency department, but many months of hospitalization and rehabilitation passed before Kayla was discharged.

The week after she returned home, Kayla picked a fight with her husband and yelled "Go to hell!" as she slammed the bedroom door. Her husband was shocked at such uncharacteristic behavior from what had once been a gentle woman. Kayla rejected hugs from family and friends who came by to see how she was doing. She got upset if anyone touched her, and at one point pushed her son away, saying, "Go away! I hate you!" Her family could not understand why Kayla, who had always been kind and circumspect in her speech, was behaving this way. Her husband wondered whether the TBI might be the cause: "She has such a short fuse these days." When Kayla announced that she was going to give away the family's beloved dog simply because the dog was getting older, her husband contacted Kayla's doctor about his concerns.

PERSONALITY CHANGES ARE NOT uncommon after TBI. In fact, the most significant problem years after a TBI may be personality changes, including increased impulsivity.

Symptoms

A person with TBI may act impulsively (acting on a whim without consideration of the consequences) or blurt out comments without weighing their effects. For example, she may criticize a family member, whereas before she would have been supportive or said nothing. She may become uncomfortably blunt and even verbally aggressive, like Kayla, above.

Impulsivity can also manifest physically. The person with TBI may be more easily upset and have a lower threshold for acting out physically. Before the TBI it may have taken a lot to upset her, but after a TBI, she may be constantly on edge and seemingly quick to lash out physically. This major change can be surprising to caregivers and family members.

Impulsivity can have significant negative consequences. For example, impulsive sexually inappropriate behavior in public can lead to legal attention, especially if directed at minors. The person with TBI may also be more likely to get into physical confrontations and indulge in her anger rather than appropriately weigh the risks, and physical and legal consequences, as she would have before her accident. Impulsive behavior can antagonize even close family members and erode support from family, as can be seen in Kayla's story. This behavior, in turn, can make it more difficult to achieve optimal recovery.

Impulsive behavior is often associated with frontal lobe injuries. The delicate location of the frontal lobes, near bony prominences of the skull, makes them particularly vulnerable to damage from violent impact. The orbitofrontal cortex, located right above the eyes, is associated with self-regulation. The orbitofrontal cortex, the anterior temporal lobes, and limbic structures (particularly the amygdala) within the temporal lobes and their connections form a neural circuit that provides impulse control. For example, frontal lobe areas such as the orbitofrontal cortex regulate the limbic system (the emotional brain). (Many of these brain structures are illustrated in figures 2.1a and b.) When the frontal lobe is damaged, a minor provocation sometimes can lead to excessive emotional response and impulsive behavior.

In some cases, impulsivity and other personality changes that arise after TBI are a magnification of tendencies that existed before the injury. Perhaps the person with TBI had been a bit impulsive. After the injury, the impulsivity may intensify, now causing distress and more serious consequences. Some have argued that people with impulsive personality traits may even be more likely to suffer traumatic brain injury to begin with because they tend to take more risks and are thus more liable to hurt themselves. But sometimes these changes occur in people who had no such personality traits before the injury, as in the case of Phineas Gage (see box, below).

Drinking alcohol and taking illicit or even some prescribed drugs are high-risk factors for sustaining TBI. Alcohol and drugs alone can make people more impulsive. Chronic or excessive use of these substances can affect the brain and lead to greater impulsivity. At the same time, these substances can make people more likely to sustain a TBI, which can exacerbate the impulsivity further, leading to

---

The Puzzling Case of Phineas Gage

The effects of frontal lobe damage were famously noted back in the nineteenth century, after an American railroad worker named Phineas Gage was hurt. Gage sustained a traumatic brain injury when a rod he was using to prepare a dynamite charge exploded, piercing his frontal lobes. He survived his injury and recovered remarkably well in most ways. However, it soon became apparent that Gage's personality had radically changed. "Gage was no longer Gage," noted a co-worker. He now spoke impulsively, was coarse and rude in his social interactions, and didn't much care how he treated others. To put it simply, he became a sociopath. Gage's case is a well-known example of what frontal lobe damage can do; there may be no obvious evidence of injury except for extreme behavioral changes such as impulsivity. People who have sustained damage to the frontal lobes can have trouble keeping their impulses in check. They may blurt out things they are thinking that they would have kept to themselves before the TBI.

a vicious cycle. People who sustain a TBI, therefore, should not drink alcohol or use drugs

Treatment

If you are concerned about impulsivity, either for yourself or for a person you care for, seek professional help. Untreated or poorly managed impulsivity has the potential to lead to unsafe or dangerous behaviors. Contact your primary care physician or a psychiatrist regarding your concerns; they will be able to help or will make appropriate referrals. Impulsivity may also be associated with other medical or emotional problems, so assessment by a professional is mandatory. In addition, psychologists or other medical professionals can administer tests to determine the nature and severity of impulsivity. Test results can help to guide treatment. Treatment of impulsivity is multipronged and includes a combination of medications, behavioral strategies, and environmental adjustments.

Environmental and Behavioral Therapies and Lifestyle Changes

Family members and caregivers of people with TBI should encourage behaviors that will help in brain recovery and decrease the incidence of impulsivity.

For example, it's helpful for the person with TBI to have a daily routine or a timetable for the day. The person with TBI should have a hand in shaping her routine and agree on the structure for her day. If you need help setting up a daily structure, ask for help from your physician or from an occupational therapist.

Minimize provocation when possible. The threshold for responding to a provocation and controlling self-regulation may be lower in people who have suffered a traumatic brain injury. Such a reduced tolerance level can lead to impulsive behaviors. Although it may be impossible to eliminate all provocation, make note and be aware of what people, comments, and situations have already led to impulsive behavior. Keep alcohol out of the house and avoid stressful topics, especially when the person with TBI appears to be less capable of self-regulation.

Help your loved one with TBI and impulsivity learn several self-regulation strategies (see "Tips for Coping," below). Breathing techniques associated with yoga, for example, can improve emotional regulation. Deep-breathing exercises and guided meditation may also be helpful in improving self-regulation.

The person with TBI benefits from some compensation for her frontal lobe deficits. Try to reduce distractors in her environment (surround her with fewer things to get impulsive about) or post reminders of useful self-regulation strategies around the house where she'll see them. Organizational aids such as calendars or schedule organizers may also be helpful so that the person with TBI knows what to do next—affording her less time or opportunity to be impulsive.

Positive reinforcement tends to work much better than punishment for people with TBI, so avoid threats and nagging. Modeling positive behavior by showing the person how to act appropriately is another way caregivers can help. Redirect the person when she acts inappropriately. Plan ahead and develop simple "impulsive-alert!" signals such as showing a time-out sign or saying a certain phrase when the person with TBI is getting impatient. One family member noted that when she finds her husband getting impatient or edgy, she tells him, "Ralph, it's time to take some deep breaths." She had already worked this out with her husband as a sign that he may be losing control and needs to calm down.

Good nutrition and adequate hydration are both important elements for successful recovery after TBI. Furthermore, omega-3 fatty acids (found in fish oil) may help with psychiatric conditions and may be helpful in TBI as well.

Drug Therapy

Some medications may help to improve frontal lobe functioning and thus decrease impulsivity. Doctors now frequently treat frontal lobe damage with amantadine, an agent originally used to treat the flu and later Parkinson's disease. It affects functioning of two neurotransmitters in the brain, dopamine and glutamate. Other medications that help impulsivity include selective serotonin re-uptake inhibitors (SSRIs) such as Lexapro (escitalopram) and Zoloft (sertraline). Tegretol (carbamazepine) is an antiseizure medicine that may also be helpful, as may Depakote (valproic acid).

In summary, traumatic brain injury can easily affect the frontal lobes and make a person vulnerable to impulsivity. People who have frontal lobe damage can behave quite differently than they did before the injury. Caregivers and family members can strive to remember to recognize the neurological basis of such behavior change and support the person with TBI as she learns and practices self-regulation skills. Seek help and guidance from a professional trained in the effects of TBI, as impulsive behaviors (and situations in which they occur) can change from day to day.

Tips for Coping with Impulsivity after TBI

If you are experiencing impulsivity after TBI:

> Learn self-regulation strategies. Try using the "Stop, Think, and Act" rule: pause and take some time to think before you act, instead of acting first and thinking later. Learn deep-breathing techniques and use them when you have the sudden urge to do something that has had bad con-sequences in the past. Using these techniques may not come easily at first, but practice helps them become a habit.

If you know someone who is experiencing impulsivity after TBI:

> Establish rules, with consequences for inappropriate behav-ior, and follow them consistently. Try not to be punitive. Positive reinforcement (rewarding by praise when something is done appropriately or well), modeling (showing the behav-ior you want your loved one with TBI to do), and redirection (distracting her with positive or more appropriate behavior when she is doing something inappropriate) helps.

> Use codes or signals when you see the person with TBI becoming irritable or edgy. Set up these codes with her when the person is calm and able to listen and participate.

> Be alert for triggers that lead to impulsivity and avoid, minimize, or remove them.

> Don't blame yourself or the person with TBI. Your loved one may be acting out for any number of reasons that have nothing to do with you. When in doubt, get help from professionals or other family members.

> Don't take it personally. Try not to take the hurtful things the person with TBI says personally, but do not accept them completely. As a family, determine acceptable behavior versus inappropriate behavior. Some behavior may be inconvenient or embarrassing, but otherwise safe. In these cases, tolerating the behavior may be the best approach.

12

Sleep Disturbances

Laura, 16, slipped and fell when she tried roller-skating for the first time and suffered a moderate TBI when her head hit the curb. She has been sleeping poorly since she left the hospital. She falls asleep easily but has trouble sleeping through the night. She wakes up early in the morning, long before she has to, and has trouble getting back to sleep before her alarm goes off. When her doctor asked about other problems, Laura admitted she wasn't enjoying things the way she used to and just wasn't motivated to do much. She also noted that it didn't take much to make her burst into tears.

Dean, 44, suffered a severe TBI when a tornado drove a tree through the front door, knocking him over as he ran for cover. He was in the hospital for three weeks, and then moved to rehabilitation. Bleeding in the brain and brain swelling complicated his medical recovery. Part of his treatment involved taking steroids. Since the brain injury, he has gained about 30 pounds. Now that he is back at home, he feels tired all day. He has also noticed that it is much harder for him to concentrate. His wife adds that Dean "snores like a freight train." His loud snoring keeps her awake at night.

Melanie, 35, sustained a TBI after she slipped in the bathroom and hit her head against the sink. Now she can't get to sleep until two in the morning and repeatedly sleeps through her alarm, waking up around ten. This insomnia has been frustrating for her because she has to report for work by eight.

SLEEP IS AN ESSENTIAL part of life. We all know this intuitively, as we often "don't feel right" or feel slower when we haven't had a good night's sleep. We feel tired or irritable. Words may not come to us as easily when we need them in conversation. In fact, even though scientists are not certain about the exact functions of sleep, we do know that lack of sleep interferes with emotional stability, cognitive functioning, and social and functional productivity. Healthy human beings spend about one-third of their lives in sleep, demonstrating just how important sleep must be for normal body functioning.

Traumatic brain injury often affects sleep. Sleep problems are about three times more common in people with TBI than they are in the general population. In fact, more than half of people with TBI experience sleep problems at some point during the recovery stage. Sleep problems, if undiagnosed or untreated, can make irritability, anxiety, depression, and memory and concentration problems worse and can greatly interfere with productivity and rehabilitation. The latter is important because engagement in rehabilitation is an active process that requires the person with TBI to put forth a lot of time and energy to derive the most benefit from treatment.

Several regions distributed throughout the brain control sleep. Small groups of nerve cells located at the base of the brain maintain sleep and wakefulness and connect to other regions of the brain via complex circuits. There are many types of sleep disorders, and many have overlapping symptoms. Here we discuss only the most common sleep disorders and provide basic principles for diagnosing and treating them.

Sleep problems can occur without other symptoms or can be associated with other medical conditions, such as infections or depression. Sleep disorders are often associated with pain and fatigue, which many people with TBI also experience. Sleep problems can affect people with TBI regardless of how severe the injury is and can occur at any point during recovery.

The Stages of Sleep

Sleep is an active brain process consisting of two basic states: rapid eye movement (REM) sleep and nonrapid eye movement (NREM) sleep. NREM sleep consists of four stages, each of which lasts between 5 and 15 minutes. In normal sleep, then, we go through five sleep stages. The stages can be differentiated by the electrical brain waves they produce, which differ in amplitude (size) and frequency (number per second). These five stages combined last a total of 90–100 minutes. People progress through a few such cycles during every normal sleep period. We recognize that shift workers often get their restorative sleep during daylight hours, but for the purposes of this discussion, we use "a good night's sleep" and similar terminology to refer to a standard episode of seven or eight hours of sleep.

Sleep thus consists of alternating stages of NREM and REM sleep. NREM sleep predominates in the early part of the night. Four or five REM periods occur in a given night's sleep, each period longer than the previous one. REM sleep accounts for about a quarter of the total sleep time; in other words, we spend about two hours per night in REM sleep.

A structure at the base of the brain called the pons activates REM sleep. The pons relays signals to the thalamus, which screens the signals and then sends them to the cortex (the outer layer of the brain, responsible for thinking and planning).

The pons also sends signals to the spinal cord that temporarily paralyze the muscles. In some ways this paralysis is a protective strategy, which prevents us from moving our limbs and acting out our dreams. In some people, this suppression does not occur, and they act out during dreaming. For example, someone who is dreaming about being attacked may thrash his hands and legs and even get out of bed, boxing and punching his "attackers." Some people have even hurt themselves while dreaming. This type of sleep abnormality is called REM sleep behavior disorder.

About three-quarters of the time that we are asleep, we are in NREM sleep. Deep NREM sleep occurs in the first part of the night. Structures in the hypothalamus control NREM sleep. Other regions, including the thalamus and the reticular activating system (RAS), are also involved.

Infants spend about half their sleeping time in REM sleep, whereas adults spend less than a quarter of total sleep time in REM. Also, as we age, the time spent in stages three and four of the NREM sleep decline. As a result, older adults have predominantly stages one and two of NREM sleep.

Causes of Sleep Disorders

Sleep problems can be the direct consequences of the brain injury itself or can result from environmental, physiological, or psychological factors. Because the most common type of brain injury is diffuse axonal injury (affecting those nerve fibers that connect different parts of the brain), and because sleep is controlled by several regions throughout the brain, it is not surprising that sleep disturbance is a common consequence of brain injury. In addition, damage to the internal biological clock in the brain that controls sleep and wakefulness (called the suprachiasmatic nucleus) can alter sleep timing. TBI may also affect regions of the brain that maintain breathing, resulting in sleep-disordered breathing, called apnea. Apnea is a marked slowing or temporary cessation of breathing, which markedly decreases the oxygen supply to the brain. Finally, chemicals in the brain that maintain sleep and wakefulness (including serotonin, norepinephrine, and acetylcholine) are also disturbed in TBI and contribute to sleep-wake disturbances.

Environmental conditions such as noise, stimulation, and bright lights are often associated with sleep problems. There is a bidirectional relationship between sleep and such factors as stress, anxiety, and depression: sleep disturbance can both precipitate these conditions and result from them. Although alcohol can help people get to sleep, it interferes with staying asleep. Medical conditions that cause cardiac and respiratory symptoms can also cause sleep disturbances or make them worse. Many medications can interfere with the sleep-wake cycle. Most over-the-counter medications and sleep aids contain antihistamines, which cause drowsiness, but they also cause dry mouth, trouble urinating, and constipation. Because these side effects can be a source of distress, interfere with memory, and further worsen sleep, it is best to avoid these medications.

Common Sleep Disorders

Laura, Dean, and Melanie in our opening stories represent the most common types of sleep disturbances, but there are many others. All sleep disorders fall into one of four common categories: sleeplessness (insomnia), excessive daytime sleepiness, sleep-disordered breathing (sleep apnea), and sleep-timing disorders (circadian rhythm disorders).

Insomnia. Insomnia is the inability to fall asleep or stay asleep. Insomnia is categorized as early, middle, or late insomnia. Early insomnia is trouble getting to sleep, middle insomnia is waking up and not being able to go back to sleep easily, and late insomnia is waking up earlier than needed and not being able to go back to sleep. All three forms of insomnia may be present in the same person, and all interfere with productivity. Late insomnia is usually associated with clinical depression. Some research suggests that insomnia is more common in the first few weeks after TBI.

Laura, in one of our opening stories, has both middle and late insomnia. She also has symptoms of clinical depression (crying spells, lack of motivation, and lack of interest), so it is quite likely that the depression is causing her to wake up too early in the morning. The depression could be related to environmental factors (the brain injury has severely impacted her life), genetic factors (a family history of depression), direct effects of the brain injury on chemicals that regulate mood, or any combination of these.

Daytime sleepiness. Drowsiness during the day is also common after TBI. A comprehensive evaluation and overnight sleep study (described below) can be helpful in distinguishing the different causes for this problem. A correct diagnosis is important because the treatment depends on the cause. Two common causes of daytime sleepiness are sleep apnea (discussed below) and narcolepsy. Narcolepsy is a condition in which the person experiences episodes of sudden and uncontrollable sleep. Although narcolepsy is typically a genetic condition (or is perhaps caused by infection), there are reports of narcolepsy after TBI. *Posttraumatic hypersomnia* refers to excessive daytime sleepiness. This term is sometimes used as an umbrella term that includes all forms of excessive daytime sleepiness or to describe posttraumatic daytime drowsiness in the absence of sleep apnea or narcolepsy. A sleep specialist can diagnose all these conditions in a sleep laboratory.

Sleep apnea. A condition of abnormal breathing, sleep apnea has three forms: obstructive, central, and mixed. With any of these types, brief pauses (up to 20 or 30 seconds) in breathing reduce the oxygen supply to the brain. The reduced oxygen leads to sudden and frequent awakening from sleep, which in turn results in daytime drowsiness. Obstructive and mixed sleep apneas also involve frequent and loud snoring, which can be bothersome and frustrating to the bed partner. Other common factors associated with sleep apnea include being overweight or obese and having a family history of apnea.

It is possible that Dean, in our opening stories, has sleep apnea. He is snoring loudly and has excessive daytime sleepiness. A sleep study would confirm or rule out this diagnosis. His weight gain could be the reason for his sleep apnea. He may have gained weight because of the steroid treatment for the brain injury or because he couldn't exercise, as he used to do, while he was recovering. The sleep apnea could also be related to direct effects of the brain injury, including damage to areas of the brain that regulate proper breathing during sleep. A sleep study will contribute to a proper diagnosis and thus to appropriate treatment.

Circadian rhythm disorders. Circadian rhythm disorders are sleep-timing disorders. We all have certain patterns to our sleep, which vary from person to person. A person's circadian rhythm reflects when that person is most awake and when they sleep. Circadian rhythm disorders are broadly categorized as either delayed sleep phase syndrome or advanced sleep phase syndrome. In both types of circadian rhythm disorder, the duration of sleep may not change, but the timing differs: going to sleep very late (delayed phase) or very early (advanced phase).

Melanie, in our opening stories, is an example of someone with a circadian rhythm disorder, delayed sleep phase syndrome. She has a tendency to sleep late, but is still able to sleep eight hours, waking up around 10 a.m. The causes of circadian rhythm disorders could be brain injury disrupting the biological clock, the person's environment (for example, exposure to excessive stimulation or light at night), or genetic influences. Unfortunately, Melanie's work schedule is such that she has to get up early in the morning. In addition to getting traditional therapy for her condition, Melanie might consider changing to a job that would allow her to start work later in the day.

Other sleep disorders. Other types of sleep problems include periodic limb movement disorder. Leg movements during sleep are not unusual, but uncontrollable and involuntary leg movements during sleep are often problematic. Restless legs syndrome (RLS) is a condition of painful creeping, crawling sensations in the legs that occurs when the person is lying down. These sensations interfere with sleep at night and cause drowsiness and fatigue during the day. Iron deficiency anemia and chronic renal failure can worsen RLS. Sleepwalking, as the name suggests, is walking or moving around during sleep or even doing some activity (eating or sitting up in bed, for example) while being unaware of doing so.

Diagnosis

Physicians who have expertise in sleep disorders are most qualified to diagnose a sleep disorder. Diagnosis usually requires a clinical evaluation and an overnight sleep test called polysomnography (PSG). Evaluations that include PSG or some other sleep study usually take place at night, but they can be performed during the day for people with circadian rhythm disorders or narcolepsy and for shift workers. In PSG, a technician applies electrodes to different parts of the patient's head and body. The electrodes feed into a central box, which in turn connects to a computer that records and stores the data. PSG measures not only electrical activity in the brain during sleep but also eye and body movements. PSG also records the duration of sleep, number of awakenings, and periods of REM and NREM sleep, all of which contribute to the diagnosis of conditions such as sleep apnea, narcolepsy, periodic leg movements, or RLS.

Treatment

The initial step in the treatment of sleep disorders is a comprehensive evaluation by a physician, which includes obtaining a general medical and psychiatric history, reviewing medications, and reviewing the patient's daytime schedule and bedtime routine. The doctor may also order an overnight sleep test to obtain objective data regarding the nature of the sleep disturbance. Based on all these results, the doctor will create a specific treatment plan.

Treatment of sleep disturbances depends on the cause. Below are treatment strategies for several common sleep conditions.

Mood or emotional issues. If sleep disturbance is secondary to depression or other psychiatric disorders, evaluation and follow-up with a psychiatrist will be necessary, as treatment should focus on medications and psychotherapy appropriate for that disorder.

Sleep apnea. Primary treatment strategies include losing weight and quitting smoking. If either of these fails, the doctor may recommend using a device that opens the airway. If you are concerned about sleep apnea for yourself or the person you are caring for, make an appointment with a specialist in sleep medicine, who can do the evaluation and provide treatment. The person with sleep apnea may benefit from a device specifically designed to open the airways during sleep.

Circadian rhythm disorders. Exposure to bright light during strategic times during the day for specific periods of time helps restore circadian rhythms and promote sleep. Bright-light therapy uses a special light box that produces more light than indoor lighting. To be effective, the intensity of bright light should be about 10,000 lux (a measurement of light intensity). Bright-light therapy in the evenings is useful for advanced sleep phase syndrome and in the mornings for delayed sleep phase syndrome. Individuals differ, and bright-light therapy should be individualized and used only as recommended by a physician. There are many types of light therapy, and inappropriate exposure to light can have negative consequences.

Melatonin is a natural hormone that controls our sleep-wake cycles. The doctor may prescribe an appropriate dosage of melatonin to help the person fall asleep earlier. Clinicians who can evaluate and treat circadian rhythm disorders include primary care doctors, psychiatrists, neurologists, psychologists, and behavioral therapists with expertise in sleep disorders.

Drug Therapy

If the doctor is not able to identify a primary cause of sleep disturbance, he or she can recommend medications that can help with sleep. The doctor will choose medications based on the person's medical and psychiatric history. The medication should help the person sleep but not cause daytime sedation, cognitive problems, or behavioral side effects. They include medications to help with getting to sleep, like trazodone, Ambien (zolpidem), Lunesta (eszopiclone), or Rozerem (a derivative of melatonin). It is best to avoid medications if possible, especially medications like Ambien and Lunesta, and to focus instead on sleep hygiene.

However, medications may be necessary in some cases. But even when medications are recommended, they should be used for the shortest time possible, ideally not more than a few days to a couple of weeks. Avoid using benzodiazepines, like Xanax (alprazolam), Klonopin (clonazepam), Valium (diazepam), or Ativan (lorazepam), to help with sleep. People taking such drugs regularly can build up a tolerance to them, and they can be addictive.

Environmental Therapy and Lifestyle Changes

Treating sleep disturbances always includes making environmental modifications and lifestyle changes. Nonmedication strategies include practicing sleep hygiene, muscle relaxation, deep-breathing techniques, imagery, and cognitive therapy, which aims to substitute realistic thoughts for inappropriate thoughts and beliefs that contribute to sleeplessness. It is best to work with a professional therapist who will be able to advise and guide you on the use of nonmedication treatment strategies.

In summary, proper sleep may be a big factor in successful recovery from traumatic brain injury. Caregivers of people with TBI must understand just how critical sleep is. Unfortunately, the brain injury itself or factors related to the brain injury can make sleep worse. As we have discussed in this chapter, structuring the environment to be more conducive to sleep is an important first step. If that is not enough, work with the doctor treating the person with TBI to identify the underlying cause or causes of the sleep disturbance, which could be many things: anxious or depressive thoughts keeping the person with TBI awake, medications the person is taking, new-onset narcolepsy or sleep apnea, disrupted normal sleep habits, or a number of other factors.

Sleep Hygiene: Tips for a Good Night's Sleep

> Maintain structure during the day. Try to establish a routine or a timetable, as this helps sleep get regulated. People with TBI, in particular, may need to set an even more rigid schedule, one that sets a specific time for getting up and going to bed every day.
> Get involved in hobbies and pleasurable activities. Engage in outdoor activities, as exposure to natural sunlight is important for maintenance of wakefulness.
> Exercise regularly. Do strenuous exercises such as jogging or aerobics in the morning and light exercises such as stretching or yoga during the evening. It is best to avoid exercising a few hours before you would like to sleep.
> Avoid daytime naps. If you must nap, limit your nap to no more than 20 to 30 minutes and try to do this around the same time every day. In other words, put the nap time on your timetable.
> Maintain a comfortable ambience in your bedroom. Set the temperature to numbers that you are most comfortable with. Cooler temperatures are better for sleep. Minimize noise and light.
> Avoid coffee, tobacco, or any other stimulants after noon.
> Use the bed only for sleep and physical intimacy. Avoid other activities, such as reading, talking, watching TV, or using electronic devices such as tablets or cell phones while

you are in bed. The mere fact of doing these activities in bed can disrupt sleep. What's more, the background light of electronic devices can make sleep more difficult to achieve.

> Keep your bedroom stress-free. Don't use your bed as an office. Avoid working on the computer or laptop, paying bills, or doing job-related paperwork.

> Have dinner at least two hours before bedtime. A late dinner can lead to acid reflux, which can affect sleep.

> Avoid over-the-counter sleep medicines or any other nonprescribed medicines.

> Avoid alcohol and illicit drugs. Although alcohol may help you *fall* asleep, it may inhibit your ability to *stay* asleep or to sleep well. It's best to avoid alcohol or illicit drugs while trying to overcome sleep disturbance.

> Don't watch the clock. Turn your alarm clock around when you are trying to sleep. Checking your cell phone or looking at the clock to see what time it is when you're trying to fall asleep can make you more anxious and make it harder to sleep.

> If you can't sleep, get out of bed. If you can't fall asleep within a reasonable amount of time in bed, get up, go to another room, and do something boring for you until you feel sleepy. At that time, go back to bed and try to sleep. If you still can't sleep after a reasonable time, then leave the room again and repeat the process described above. Do this as many times as necessary until you fall asleep. The idea here is that you want your mind to associate the bed with sleeping, not with *not* sleeping. The greater percentage of the time that you are sleeping while in bed, the easier it will be to get to sleep when in bed.

> Consult a specialist. If sleep problems persist, have your doctor refer you to a physician with expertise in sleep disorders; a thorough evaluation, including sleep studies, can help in establishing the diagnosis. The diagnosis will determine the appropriate treatment.

PART IV

Cognitive Problems Caused by the Traumatized Brain

Cognitive problems frequently linger after traumatic brain injury, often in people who have moderate to severe brain injury, but even in those with repetitive mild injuries. By *cognitive* we refer to our ability to think, remember, and plan—that is, the abilities that are critical to our sense of self, of who we are.

The kind of cognitive impairment after TBI can be a mix of attention, memory, and other higher-order functions. We open the cognitive section of this book with attention problems occurring after TBI because we consider attention the gateway to other cognitive functions. We then discuss memory, executive function, and language.

13

Attention

Michael is a busy 41-year-old lawyer with his own law practice in a small town on Lake Erie. He sustained a moderate TBI in a boating accident one weekend. Although he was a bit banged up, he recovered well enough to return to work just two weeks after the accident. Before the TBI, Michael prided himself on his ability to multitask and get things done—his practice and his clients depended on it. Now, several months after the TBI, he admits that he feels a lot slower; he reluctantly turned over two big cases to his law partner because he feared he wouldn't perform well in court. These days he keeps his office door closed so that he can really concentrate; he finds it supremely hard to focus when there are distractions in the hallway and outer office. "Any little noise bothers me. I just can't focus," he says.

ATTENTION IS A COMMONLY USED word whose meaning we all have an intuitive sense about. In a more scientific sense, attention involves the ability to focus and choose something from a number of stimuli. At some point, we have all been told or told others to "pay attention." Without paying attention, it is hard to remember things or manipulate information or reach our goals.

Despite our intuitive sense of its meaning, attention is not one single phenomenon. There are three distinct forms of attention: selective attention, sustained attention, and divided attention. On a more fundamental level, we can think of arousal, the state of wakefulness that allows us to interact with the environment, as a form of attention, too.

How TBI Affects Attention

The person with TBI can experience a range of arousal states, from coma to hyperarousal (agitation). Impaired arousal generally occurs immediately after the brain injury, and the person becomes more alert as he gradually recovers. People with TBI can have problems with one or several subtypes of attention, from problems with arousal alone or compounded by deficits in selective, sustained, or divided attention.

As people with TBI recover, they may pass through a phase of delirium, itself an attention disorder. People in a state of delirium cannot focus or sustain their attention for significant periods. Confusion and disorientation in this state can trigger agitation or even aggression. The delirium must resolve for a person to recover from TBI, but difficulties with selective attention and sustained attention persist for many people.

Selective attention is the mechanism by which the brain chooses which stimuli in the environment to engage with. It involves the ability to inhibit or ignore the processing of distractions. When we think about paying attention or being distracted, we are usually referring to selective attention.

Sustained attention or vigilance, refers to maintaining focus on something for a longer time than is required for selective attention. People with TBI may have trouble keeping their focus for more than a brief period, perhaps just seconds. As recovery occurs, both selective and sustained attentions tend to improve. Selective and sustained attention impairments usually occur in moderate to severe TBI.

Divided attention is the ability to maintain focus on more than one task at a time. It reflects an ability to supervise aspects of attention because it involves switching between tasks and monitoring the attentional system. Divided attention is one component of executive function (see Chapter 15). Divided attention difficulties can occur at all levels of TBI severity. People with even mild TBI can feel subjectively that they can no longer multitask efficiently. Problems with divided attention may persist in those with moderate to severe TBI, affecting day-to-day functioning, as illustrated in Michael's story, above. Many people with TBI who are struggling with divided attention complain that they have difficulty multitasking.

Attention is critical for other cognitive functions because we need attention to store things into memory. Once in memory, we can manipulate information and act on our goals. Because attention is such a basic and critical function, it depends upon diffuse neural circuits throughout the brain. This arrangement is both good and bad. This built-in redundancy makes attention more resilient than other cognitive functions and therefore more quickly recoverable. On the other hand, because the circuits controlling attention are spread throughout the brain, a wide range of brain injuries can have an impact on attention.

Arousal, our baseline attention level, is housed at the back of the brain in the brainstem, which connects the spinal cord to the rest of the brain. The reticular formation is the circuit in the brainstem that is critical in maintaining our ability to attend at all and that controls arousal. Damage to this reticular formation can result in coma.

Selective attention involves a diffuse circuit that includes the posterior parietal lobe, the dorsolateral prefrontal cortex, and the anterior cingulate, along with the thalamus and basal ganglia. The thalamus, basal ganglia, and parietal lobe supply different types of input to the rest of the selective attention circuit, and in doing so, guide the targets of attention. For example, the thalamus sends sensory information, the basal ganglia sends motor information, and the parietal lobe sends spatial information throughout the circuit. Such input is vital because the selective attentional circuit needs to know where the sensory stimulus is that we have to attend to, and then where the target is that we have to respond to by moving our limbs. The dorsolateral prefrontal cortex and anterior cingulate are thought to utilize all this information to ultimately do the "selecting" of selective attention—that is, selecting to attend to something. (These parts of the brain are illustrated in figures 2.1a and b.)

Sustained attention, or vigilance, may be encoded by a particular part of the brainstem and its influence over the right hemisphere of the brain. Divided attention may be related to other, even more diffuse, networks in the brain controlled by the white matter tracts connecting different parts of the brain.

Treatment
Environmental and Behavioral Therapies
and Lifestyle Changes

Impaired attention benefits from both environmental and behavioral interventions. As a caregiver or family member of a person who has suffered a traumatic brain injury, you can help by eliminating sources of distraction, particularly overstimulation. Because a person with impaired attention has trouble distinguishing between what he should pay attention to and what he should not, he may get overwhelmed and fatigued if there are too many people or too many things going on around him. His inability to process overstimulation can also lead to irritability and agitation.

The person with TBI who has attention problems can benefit greatly from having a predictable schedule. Plan activities that require significant attention and effort for times when he is rested. Sleep is thus a particularly critical factor in recovery. A person with TBI who is not sleeping well will likely have trouble focusing his attention. (See Chapter 12 for information about sleep disturbances and treatment for sleep disturbances.)

Cognitive rehabilitation is a formal approach to teaching cognitive skills and providing exercises to practice them. Attention training immediately after the TBI is usually unnecessary because in most cases attention improves spontaneously as the brain recovers. During rehabilitation, however, whether in the rehabilitation hospital or at home, attention training can be helpful, and is best done with supervision and guidance from a clinician, such as an occupational therapist or a speech-language therapist. Computer-based attention-training programs may be useful, although they are best done in conjunction with a clinician. In addition, people like Michael in our opening story may benefit from vocational rehabilitation programs, which provide a range of services, from job analysis and career counseling to case management and psychosocial interventions, that can help people return to work and maintain their job.

Drug Therapy

Medications may also play a role in treating attention deficits after TBI. They should be used only as prescribed by a doctor. Self-adjustment or self-prescription can be dangerous and harmful, as these medications can lead to unwanted changes in heart rate or blood pressure.

Amantadine, an agent that acts on glutamate and dopamine, may help recovery of arousal. Other helpful medications include agents that increase dopamine and norepinephrine (stimulants) and agents that increase acetylcholine. Stimulants like Ritalin (methylphenidate) and Adderall (dextroamphetamine) can help with various aspects of attention. They can support arousal and improve sustained attention.

Acetylcholinesterase inhibitors like Aricept (donepezil) can also help with attention. These agents, however, are not as specific to attention as are stimulants. Although they can help a range of cognitive difficulties, they may be particularly helpful in controlling divided attention, as opposed to selective or sustained attention.

In summary, attention is a critical aspect of cognition because it is the gateway to other cognitive functions. Because circuits throughout the brain control attention, traumatic brain injury frequently affects attention. Problems with attention usually resolve, but it may remain difficult for a person with TBI to comprehend things as well as he did before the injury.

Tips for Coping with Attention Problems after TBI
If you are experiencing attention problems after TBI:

> Establish structure and routine for the day. Try to maintain the same routine.
> Minimize distraction. Simple things like turning off the radio while driving or switching off the TV while having a conversation cut down on distractions immensely. Electronic devices like smart phones or tablets or social media networks can add exponentially to the attentional burden, so it's best to avoid them for the time being.

> Maintain adequate sleep to make sure you get enough rest. Lack of sleep, poor quality of sleep, or sleep disorders (see Chapter 12) could be a major cause of attention problems after TBI.

> Take your time to complete a task, focusing on one aspect at a time. If necessary, break each task down into smaller steps.

> Consult your doctor if you are a student and are having trouble keeping up with school work or meeting deadlines. Your doctor can determine whether you will benefit from certain accommodations at school.

> It is possible that you may have underlying ADHD (attention deficit hyperactivity disorder) that was not previously diagnosed and has perhaps been made worse by the TBI. Consider seeing a physician who specializes in attentional disorders to look into this possibility.

> Computerized brain-training programs may help leverage the brain's plasticity—its ability to use new pathways after injury. These programs can help with attention, but they should be used under the supervision and guidance of a clinician. To maximize recovery, follow these brain-training programs regularly. Frequency and consistency are key; doing the exercises just once in a while is ineffective.

> Any one of these strategies by itself may not work. A holistic approach, that combines a variety of strategies, is often necessary.

14

Memory

A car struck Roseanne's car from behind on an icy road, and Roseanne's head banged hard again her windshield as she slid into a snowbank. Roseanne sat in her front seat, disoriented, for about 20 minutes, until the ambulance arrived to take her to the nearest hospital. In the emergency department, doctors diagnosed Roseanne with traumatic brain injury from contusions in the right and left frontotemporal regions of the brain; in other words, she had multiple bruises on the front and sides of her brain. She was admitted to the hospital for observation and monitoring, and discharged several days later.

Physically, Roseanne recovered quickly, but she noticed at once that things were harder to remember than they had been. In her first week back at home, she misplaced her cell phone many times, left the tea kettle boiling on the stove, and had to look up her husband's work number every time she wanted to call him. Two weeks after the accident, she started to feel hurt that her sister hadn't called to check on her, until her husband reminded her that her sister had called twice in the past week. Over the next few months, Roseanne grew more and more frustrated at her inability to remember things. She tried making notes about what she had to do—doctor's appointment, shopping lists—but then she forgot about the notes: "I have to write notes all the time but then I forget where I put my notes!" After Roseanne missed a third follow-up appointment with her neurologist, the doctor began to suspect that his 55-year-old patient was having serious repercussions from the TBI, and he called her husband, who brought her in the next day.

MEMORY PROBLEMS DEVELOP in many people after traumatic brain injury. Although this chapter focuses on memory difficulties, memory problems often occur together with other cognitive deficits, particularly impaired attention. For example, if we are not able to pay attention to information, we are not likely to remember it. Also, considering that TBI is a diffuse process that can affect much of the brain (and the connections between different parts of the brain), "memory" problems may reflect damage to multiple parts of the brain, which means that multiple, distinct cognitive deficits occur together.

Memory is not a single, unitary cognitive function, despite our intuition that it is one thing. We have an intuitive sense of what memory is and what it is like not to remember, but in the brain, memory is housed in different neural circuits, and there are different types of memory.

Memory is a collection of processes that lead to learning and recalling information. There are two kinds of memory: explicit memory and implicit memory. Explicit memory is what we typically think of as memory—information we must consciously make an effort to remember, for example, remembering what someone told us a few minutes ago, what we ate for breakfast yesterday, or what movie we saw last week. Implicit memory is more subtle. Implicit memory is information we remember without consciously trying to: how to walk, or eat with a fork, or ride a bicycle.

Explicit memory, in turn, can be either episodic or semantic. Episodic memory remembers personal events, like what happened at work yesterday or who came by for dinner tonight. Semantic memory remembers facts we learned in the past, for example, cars have four tires or the blue whale is the largest animal.

TBI mostly affects episodic memory. In most cases, the more severe the brain injury, the worse the episodic memory. Damage to episodic memory is what most caregivers of people with TBI notice and struggle with. A good example of having an episodic memory problem is Roseanne's symptoms, in our opening story. She couldn't remember conversations she had had with family and colleagues, and she often forgot where she had left her cell phone.

A person with brain injury, too, may forget within minutes what she has been told to do. It may seem that she is ignoring what you told her, but it could well be that she has a deficit in episodic memory and simply doesn't remember what you said. Episodic memory is also the type of memory most affected by Alzheimer's disease. Alzheimer's disease attacks areas of the brain that house episodic memory; TBI may damage those very same areas.

Traumatic brain injury does not appear to affect implicit memory and semantic memory as much as it affects episodic memory. TBI can affect other aspects of memory, such as working memory and metamemory. Working memory is the ability to remember things for a few seconds and then manipulate and use that information. You hear a phone number on the radio, you memorize it, and then you call the number using your cell phone—that's working memory. Metamemory is memory of memory, that is, awareness of one's own memory. Deficits in metamemory can lead people with TBI to deny they have any memory problems at all, which can lead to resistance to rehabilitation and to well-meaning suggestions from family or caregivers.

As we mentioned earlier, memory is closely tied to attention. To remember something, we first need to pay attention. Working memory is an extension of our attentional system, letting us pay attention long enough to put things into memory. Working memory allows us to keep something (an idea, an image, a telephone number) in our brain for a few seconds before the brain stores it in short-term memory (which lasts minutes). The brain then transfers short-term memory to long-term memory. TBI tends to impact working memory and short-term memory more than long-term memory.

To remember something, then, we have to pay attention (use working memory) long enough to store the information in short-term memory and then transfer the short-term memory into long-term storage. We then have to be able to retrieve the information from memory. TBI can affect all these aspects of memory, depending on where the brain damage is.

Memory assessment is an integral part of assessing the severity of TBI. The phrase *posttraumatic amnesia* refers to how long it takes a person with TBI to be able to remember new information. The longer the period of posttraumatic amnesia, the worse the brain injury is considered to be.

The neural circuitry of memory lies at least in part in two areas of the brain: the inner (medial) side of the temporal lobe, which includes the hippocampus, and the upper outer surface of the frontal lobe, known as the dorsolateral prefrontal cortex. Unfortunately, the temporal and frontal lobes are both particularly vulnerable to brain trauma and are often damaged in TBI.

The medial temporal lobe circuit is important in episodic, short-term memory; it stores information that we have just learned, perhaps what someone said to us a few minutes ago. Of course, for information to get into short-term memory, the attentional system (which has networks across much of the brain) must send the information to the memory system. The attentional system first sends the information to the working memory system, which is housed in the frontal lobe. The frontal lobe sends that information to the medial temporal lobe for short-term storage. Eventually, information from short-term memory is distributed to various locations throughout the brain for long-term storage. Visual long-term information goes to visual areas; long-term auditory memories go to auditory areas, and so on. The frontal lobe has a critical role in organizing memories and permitting appropriate access and retrieval.

So, what seems like an automatic process—remembering what someone asked us to do a few minutes ago—involves the proper functioning of multiple areas of the brain. Normally, we do this quickly and automatically, but traumatic brain injury can cause difficulty at multiple steps of the process. The person with TBI may have trouble with working memory, so she can't keep the information around long enough to store it. If she can store the information in short-term memory, she may have trouble organizing the information. Even if that mechanism is intact, she may not be able to retrieve the information quickly and accurately.

Treatment

Treatment for memory problems after TBI does not usually rely on medications, although medications are available that may help. In cases of mild TBI, the keys are adequate rest and education about the recovery process. Most people with mild TBI recover their memory capabilities spontaneously, without treatment or rehabilitation. They can form new memories within 24 hours after the injury. Full recovery, as defined by the ability to organize new memories and retrieve them as efficiently as before, can take up to three months. The person must avoid additional TBIs during recovery. For example, many current guidelines now recommend that anyone who sustains a mild TBI while playing sports should come out of the game immediately. This advice is partly to avoid further TBIs, which could complicate the recovery process.

Recognizing the problem is the first step in helping with the problem. Caregivers or family members may not realize that the person with brain injury is having difficulty learning and remembering new information and may blame her for not following instructions or for being careless. During rehabilitation, family and caregivers should work with their loved one with TBI and memory problems to manage her expectations and advocate patience.

Environmental and Behavioral Therapies and Lifestyle Changes

At home, building structure into the day and minimizing distractions improves memory function. Avoiding overstimulation can help. Having a predictable schedule for sleeping, waking up, taking meals, working, and other activities can make more things automatic, so the brain doesn't have to work so hard. Protecting the brain from becoming overtaxed can in turn be helpful in recovery. Keeping things in the same place all the time can help your loved one stop misplacing items. These steps maximize the chances of success and increase confidence for the person with TBI.

Have the person with TBI and memory problems do the most taxing tasks of the day at a time when she is most rested. Build rest breaks into the day. Fatigue can be a significant issue with TBI, so minimize fatigue as much as possible to maximize memory performance. Make visitors and guests aware that they should not disrupt your loved one's rest time or schedule.

Cognitive "prosthetics," such as notebooks, cell phones, tablets, calendars, and other devices, can cue memory. Not only can these items provide reminders when needed but, more importantly, they can also reassure the person, allowing her to worry less about having to remember. Relieving her of this responsibility lets her relax and, paradoxically, may help her remember better.

Cognitive rehabilitation with a professional therapist teaches strategies to improve memory and to set up the environment in ways that enhance memory performance. One of the challenges for the person with TBI is to generalize what she learns in a formal cognitive rehabilitation setting to home. Therefore, one of the goals of the training is to make things more automatic and allow the person with TBI to learn to apply what she has learned to daily life.

Drug Therapy

Medications to improve memory are a supplement to the techniques discussed above. However, in some cases they are necessary, particularly in moderate to severe TBI. Two classes of medications may be helpful: those that increase the neurotransmitter acetylcholine and those that boost the effects of the neurotransmitters dopamine and norepinephrine.

Aricept (donepezil), Exelon (rivastigmine), and Reminyl (galantamine) are medications that increase acetylcholine. All three are also used to treat Alzheimer's disease. The research studies of the use of these medications in TBI show mixed results, but in our experience, these drugs may help improve memory in some people. Aricept is used most often, but there is no evidence that one drug is more effective than another.

Agents that increase dopamine and norepinephrine can lead to cognitive improvements. They include Ritalin (methylphenidate) and Adderall (dextroamphetamine), agents often used to treat attention deficit hyperactivity disorder. An advantage of these medications is that they are quick acting and may improve attention and processing speed and thus improve memory indirectly. Studies of these medications in TBI generally show some cognitive benefit.

Amantadine is a medication that was originally used to treat the flu and is still used occasionally to treat Parkinson's disease. It affects dopamine and another neurotransmitter, glutamate. Some studies indicate that amantadine may help with some cognitive processes, mostly attention, processing speed, and executive functioning. As we have discussed, these other cognitive functions may affect memory as well. Amantadine may thus indirectly improve memory. Namenda (memantine), a derivative of amantadine, is used to treat Alzheimer's disease and may enhance overall cognitive function.

Drugs that work primarily to increase dopamine, such as levodopa, selegiline, and bromocriptine, may be helpful in some people with TBI.

Certain antidepressants may also be helpful in treating memory problems, especially if there are also additional symptoms of clinical depression. However, the data supporting a benefit from these agents is weaker than for the mainstays of cognitive enhancement in TBI: stimulants like Ritalin and agents that increase acetylcholine, like Aricept.

In summary, memory is not one single process. There are subtypes of memory, and many other areas of cognition affect memory. Work with your loved one with TBI and memory problems and understand the frustration she faces when she tries to remember things she once knew, but that now come only with a struggle. People with TBI, especially mild TBI, do recover. Because our brains normally change all the time—in a process referred to as "plasticity"—every time we learn something new, the capacity to recover is built in. Supporting the person with TBI and memory problems as she goes through rehabilitation, helping her structure her days, and encouraging her to follow her doctors' advice and take her medications as prescribed will all help her greatly in her recovery.

Tips for Coping with Memory Problems after TBI

If you are experiencing memory problems after TBI:

> "A place for everything, and everything in its place." Make sure there is a place for everything and keep things in the same place every time. Consistent organization like this may help you to stop misplacing items and can cut down on unnecessary frustration.

> Use external devices such as notebooks, cell phones, tablets, and calendars to make notes to help cue memory. Place sticky note reminders throughout the house, in key rooms like the kitchen, bedroom, family room, and bathroom, to help you remember tasks.

> If you are having difficulty working on a task because you cannot remember directions given to you, get help. In cases like this, teaming up with someone to do tasks can be enjoyable and lead to task completion.

If you know someone who is experiencing memory problems after TBI:

> "Buddy up." As a caregiver, offer your support and buddy up with the person with TBI whenever possible to complete tasks.

> Make to-do lists of things that the person with TBI has to accomplish that day.

> Consult the doctor if mood problems or physical symptoms accompany the memory problems.

15

Executive Function

Dane plummeted 150 feet to the ground while inspecting a water tower. As he fell, his safety harness spun him in circles, bouncing him against the metal scaffolding on his way down. He suffered a severe TBI and was in a coma for ten days. After the initial hospitalization, 41-year-old Dane was transferred to a recovery unit for intense rehabilitation. Despite four long weeks of arduous therapy and valiant effort, Dane was not permitted to return home after rehabilitation because he was unable to manage his own affairs. The occupational therapist (OT) evaluated Dane and declared it unsafe for him to live alone. In her report, the OT gave several examples to explain her decision: Dane could not follow the steps to write a check or fill out a simple form, so he was incapable of managing his paperwork or paying his bills. And although Dane was *physically* capable of simple activities such as making a sandwich or peeling vegetables, he had difficulty staying on task—during the OT evaluation, he fixed an omelet but walked away without switching off the stove. His medical team determined that Dane was clearly having executive function difficulties and recommended that he move to a group home for people who have suffered a traumatic brain injury.

COGNITIVE PROBLEMS ARE COMMON after TBI, as we discuss in earlier chapters. As noted before, there are several aspects of cognition, such as memory, attention, processing speed, language, and executive function, and although we separate these functions out, in reality, there is a great deal of overlap among them. In this chapter, we focus on executive function.

Executive function is the ability to plan, organize, put things in sequence, monitor whether one's behavior is leading to its goal, and modify that behavior if one is not meeting the goals. Executive function, in short, is the ability to set a goal, initiate action toward the goal, monitor progress toward the goal, and modify the course if necessary to achieve the goal.

Executive function happens mainly within the frontal lobes. Unfortunately, the frontal lobes are particularly vulnerable to TBI because the lower portions of the frontal lobe sit on the bony interior ridges of the skull and are thus likely to be injured in mechanical trauma to the head. As a consequence, executive function impairment is common in people who have suffered a traumatic brain injury. Deficits in executive function are often a critical component in the level of functioning in a person who has TBI—for example, whether the person can live independently.

There are three aspects of executive function: cognitive, motivational, and emotional. From a cognitive point of view, executive function capabilities direct other cognitive functions, such as attention, memory, language, and movement. For example, the ability to pay attention to several things at once (divided attention) depends on executive function circuitry in the brain. The executive function system has to allocate attentional resources, select an attentional target, deal with interfering information, and switch between things that need to be attended to. Working memory, the ability to manipulate information held in memory for a few seconds, is also an executive function, as is the ability to efficiently organize this information into long-term memory.

Symptoms

A person with TBI who has problems with the cognitive aspects of executive function appears to have problems with attention, memory, or reasoning. He may not be as fluent as he was before the accident. He may take longer to think of the right word. His thinking may be slower. Even a person with a mild TBI can have noticeable deficits in these areas, especially when he has to perform demanding or complex tasks. Even if he can complete the task, it takes him longer to do so, and he must put more effort into it.

Executive function is usually associated with the portions of the frontal lobes called the prefrontal lobes and their projections. Scientists believe that the cognitive aspects of executive function are associated with a part of the frontal lobe called the dorsolateral prefrontal cortex. Cognitive executive function can be impaired even without direct damage to the dorsolateral prefrontal cortex, but in such cases, the cause is usually damage to the white matter tracts that connect this part to other parts of the brain. Damage to these connecting tracts is common in TBI, especially mild TBI, even though the damage may not be evident on our usual MRI scans.

Executive function circuits also include the medial prefrontal cortex, the part of the brain responsible for motivation: setting goals, initiating action, and sustaining activity until the goal is met. Significant damage to this circuit can lead to a condition known as abulia, or lack of will to do anything. An extreme form of abulia, in which the person may not move or speak, is called akinetic mutism. Typically, however, a person with abulia is slow to complete tasks, has a decreased ability to speak fluently, and has a hard time initiating or starting a task. Scientists believe that a particular part of the medial prefrontal cortex, the anterior cingulate, is important in supervising attention and dealing with new situations. Thus, the medial prefrontal cortex helps in choosing a goal and initiating action, whereas the dorsolateral prefrontal cortex is involved in planning and monitoring the action.

Another circuit, the ventral part of the prefrontal cortex (particularly the orbitofrontal cortex), lies at the border between the cognitive and emotional parts of the brain. At this strategic location, the orbitofrontal cortex integrates emotion with cognitive function. This part of the brain is particularly vulnerable to TBI, and damage to it likely explains the deficits in real-life decision making and social functioning that are common in people with TBI. People who have damage to the ventromedial prefrontal cortex, like Phineas Gage (see Chapter 11), have trouble understanding others' feelings, being socially appropriate, and keeping their impulses in check.

We have discussed the three distinct aspects of executive function: cognitive, motivational, and emotional. But TBI often causes diffuse damage that affects multiple aspects of all these circuits. It is helpful for you as a caregiver of a person with TBI to be aware of these circuits and the behaviors that can stem from damage to these areas of the brain so that you can make sense of your loved one's behavior. He may be slower mentally than before. He may have trouble solving simple, everyday problems. He may need help to organize and plan his life. He may act inappropriately in public. It's common for a person with TBI to have a combination of some or all of these issues.

Treatment

There are things that you as a caregiver can do to help your loved one with TBI who is suffering from executive function impairment. Most important, however, is to understand that he will be slower or more disorganized or act differently than he did before the TBI, and to be patient with him.

Environmental and Behavioral Therapies and Lifestyle Changes

One woman who had a traumatic brain injury was very aware of her new situation: "I used to be the multitasking queen," she said, "but now I can only do one thing at a time." Because organizational skills are often impaired after TBI, help your loved one to get organized and stay organized. For example, he may need help organizing his office at home or keeping his calendar up to date. He may benefit from a regular schedule. Because he may have trouble planning and sequencing, help him to break small tasks down into smaller components and guide him on what to do next. Family members may need to take over bill paying or other complex tasks until the person recovers.

Cognitive rehabilitation can help retrain the brain and teach executive function skills. This type of teaching usually happens in a neurorehabilitation clinic staffed by neuropsychologists, physical therapists, speech-language therapists, and occupational therapists who are specially trained to work with people with brain injury. Depending on the nature of the injury, one or more of these experts works with the patient. Rehabilitation can involve coaching or role playing that teaches ways to improve self-regulation and overcome obstacles. The idea is to teach the person with TBI "scripts" for what to do in different situations and provide opportunities to practice the scripts. With practice, these scripts become automatic, so when the person encounters the situation in real life, he doesn't have to overtax his decision-making skills. Such training paves the way for better decision making. Cognitive rehabilitation can also focus on retraining social skills using "scripts" that teach the person with a TBI what to do when he meets a stranger, for example. A person with TBI who exhibits socially inappropriate behavior can benefit from receiving positive reinforcement (a reward or praise) when he acts appropriately in a social situation.

Drug Therapy

Medications are not the primary method of treatment for people with executive dysfunction, but some medications are indeed effective. Amantadine affects several neurotransmitters, including glutamate and dopamine, and may help people with poor executive function after TBI both cognitively and behaviorally. It may help to facilitate self-monitoring and hence improve behavior.

Acetylcholinesterase inhibitors like Aricept (donepezil) affect a neurotransmitter called acetylcholine and may help executive function in addition to their primary benefit of improving memory.

Stimulants like Ritalin (methylphenidate) and Adderall (dextroamphetamine), which affect dopamine and norepinephrine, may also be used. They clearly help with processing speed and attention, and they may improve the attentional aspects of executive function.

In summary, damage to executive function capabilities because of TBI can cause significant functional impairment. These changes can be subtle, and it may not be apparent that they are due to brain damage. People may think that the person with TBI is being stubborn or lazy or difficult. Caregivers who understand the aspects of executive dysfunction also understand that cognitive and behavioral changes after TBI may reflect brain damage and may not be deliberate. Of course, it is important to help the person with TBI regain a sense of control over his life. Encourage him to follow his doctors' advice and to actively participate in his rehabilitation. Discourage him from doing things that can make executive function worse, such as using drugs or alcohol or engaging in reckless behavior. With the support of family, people with TBI can relearn skills and accept their new baseline while improving their lives.

Tips for Coping with Executive Function Deficits after TBI

If you know someone who is experiencing executive function deficits after TBI:

> ❯ Organization is the key to stability. Remember and follow the four pillars of managing executive function deficits.
>   - Structure. Structure in all forms reduces both stress and disorganization. Keep a daily schedule, a routine, a plan that the person with TBI can count on to structure his day.
>   - Consistency. Consistency promotes learning. Consistent responses to behavior and consistent daily routines, for example, will help the person with TBI learn what is expected and what he can rely on.
>   - Timetable of activities. Keeping a timetable for daytime activities that includes built-in breaks increases engagement and reduces boredom and fatigue.
>   - Rules, with flexibility. A code of conduct needs to be maintained for the person with TBI, but it cannot be black and white—there must be opportunities for compromise. Behaviors that may appear odd or strange but are not harmful or unsafe are permissible. In other words, you don't have to fight every battle. Just fight the battles that are worth winning.
> ❯ Practice positive reinforcement: "You catch more flies with honey than you do with vinegar." Positive reinforcement in the form of reward or praise for good behavior encourages

and thus helps maintain that behavior. Merely punishing the person for behavior he can't control can lead to outbursts or rebellious behavior.

> Write and rehearse scripts for coping with stressful situations. Work with your loved one to practice what he will do in certain situations so that when the situation arises, the appropriate response comes easily.

> Seek professional help. If the person you care for is in trouble for acting out, work with professionals to explore options for helping him. Physicians, psychologists, and therapists may all be on "the team" that can help the person with executive function problems to recover.

16

Language

At age 47, Nadira sustained a moderate traumatic brain injury in a car accident. She recovered well overall and was released from rehabilitation with appointments for several follow-up visits over the next few months. Once at home, Nadira felt fine physically, but she noticed that it was hard to find the words she was looking for, both in her daily thoughts and in conversations with others.

At her first follow-up appointment, Nadira greeted the neurologist when she walked in.

"Hi, Dr. Hansen. It's nice to . . ."

Nadira paused.

". . . *look* you again," she completed, and then broke down in tears.

Nadira explained to the neurologist the trouble she had finding words, even when talking to herself.

"I hate to go out anymore," she confessed. "So many people are happy to see me after the accident, but I just can't speak properly anymore! I find myself reaching, reaching . . . and it's *just* on the tip of my tongue, but when I speak, the wrong word comes out. It's so frustrating! What is wrong with me?"

THE MEDICAL NAME for disturbance of expression and comprehension of spoken language is *aphasia*. Aphasia may also be associated with deficits in written communication (dysgraphia) or reading (dyslexia). Language has a very specific circuit in the brain, and neuroscience is familiar with this language circuit and how it functions. People with TBI can experience aphasia if the damage they suffer directly impacts the language circuit in the brain.

Symptoms

Aphasia has two fundamental forms: nonfluent aphasia and fluent aphasia. People with nonfluent aphasia have difficulty speaking. Their speech output is diminished or minimal—or nonexistent: some people become nonverbal. People with nonfluent aphasia may use only single words or short phrases. Speech is slow and effortful. Their speech may sound telegraphic, in that, like an old-fashioned telegraph, it is composed of only a word and then a pause, a word and then a pause. As in a telegraph, only the main words in a sentence, the nouns and verbs, are used, but no conjunctions, which connect words. Despite their trouble speaking, however, people with nonfluent aphasia generally remain able to comprehend speech. They can usually respond to verbal requests but cannot repeat phrases.

Fluent aphasia is characterized by deficits in understanding and comprehension. People with fluent aphasia use words that are incorrect for what they want to express. Such substitutions are called paraphasias. People with this condition are fluent, meaning that they speak at a normal rate and pronounce words correctly, but others have difficulty understanding them because what they say does not make sense. Fluent aphasia is sometimes called jargon aphasia. People with fluent aphasia often substitute one word for the other: they say *car* when they want to say *far* or *cat* when they mean to say *dog*. Many people with fluent aphasia are frustrated that others cannot understand them, but they may lack insight into their own language dysfunction. Indeed, in the past, some patients thought to have schizophrenia may have had fluent aphasia; observers may have misunderstood their language problem for psychosis.

Anomia, or difficulty in naming objects, is a form of fluent aphasia and is a common language problem in people with TBI. The person with TBI may appear to have memory problems, but what is really happening is that she is unable to find the right word.

Some people have intact fluency and comprehension but have trouble repeating phrases. Damage resulting in both fluent and non-fluent aphasia can result in global, or total aphasia.

Aprosody, another type of language problem seen in people with traumatic brain injury, is difficulty in appreciating or portraying emotions in speech. Much of what we communicate through our speech is more than just the words we speak, and much of the emotion we convey with our speech is not expressed in the words themselves. Being able to understand the emotions behind the words is an important human skill. But a person with aprosody may have difficulty understanding that when someone who is angry says, "Well, that's great!" they are being sarcastic. She may interpret the phrase literally and wonder why, in the midst of something going wrong, someone would say "that's great." In addition to difficulty in understanding the emotions associated with speech, she may also have difficulty modulating her speech and expressing her words with emotion. For example, her speech patterns may be monotonous and flat. Understandably, then, aprosody as a consequence of TBI can affect how a person with TBI interacts with her family and caregivers—a frustrating situation for all involved.

Language is one of the most localized and best understood cognitive functions in the brain. We know which areas of the brain are associated with the ability to express, comprehend, and repeat. We also know the areas of the brain associated with the ability to incorporate emotions into language. The frontal and temporal lobes house these language abilities. Although TBI usually causes diffuse brain injury, the frontal and temporal lobes are particularly vulnerable to injury.

For most people, the left hemisphere of the brain houses language and is called the dominant hemisphere for language functions. This is always the case for right-handed people (most of the population). In most left-handed people, language is housed in the left hemisphere, but less commonly than in right-handed people. That is, the language circuitry of left-handed people tends to be, to some degree, in both hemispheres—the left and the right.

Within the left dominant hemisphere, the language circuit includes Wernicke's area, in the upper temporal lobe, which controls the comprehension of spoken and written speech; Broca's area, in the lower frontal lobe, which processes information into an organized pattern necessary for verbalization; and the arcuate fasciculus, which connects Wernicke's area and Broca's area. Damage to Wernicke's area can cause fluent aphasia; damage to Broca's area can cause nonfluent aphasia; and damage to the arcuate fasciculus can cause difficulty in repeating speech, or conduction aphasia. As noted above, difficulty finding the right word is called anomia, which is a form of fluent aphasia. It results from damage to areas near Wernicke's area in the temporal lobe and the inferior parietal lobe. Anomia can also occur because of the more diffuse brain damage of the type commonly seen in TBI. Nadira's condition, in our opening story, indicates that she has anomia. A person with anomia might say, for example, that she wanted to get the *cat* out when she meant that she wanted to get the *car* out.

Other aspects of language involve different areas of the brain. The non-dominant hemisphere (the right side of the brain for most people) manages the "body language" and emotional content of speech. The non-dominant hemisphere is also responsible for cursing, likely because of the emotional aspect in cursing, so damage to the dominant hemisphere usually does not affect a person's ability to curse. It can be startling to hear someone who cannot speak more than a few words suddenly curse fluently! Finally, because singing can also reflect non-dominant hemisphere functioning, people with TBI and nonfluent aphasia may not be able to engage in normal conversation but may retain the ability to sing what they want to express.

Treatment

Without an understanding of the subtleties of language dysfunction that can develop after TBI, it is easy to misinterpret problems with language as lack of motivation and depression. Although the person with TBI may be depressed—and that possibility certainly must be considered—it is also possible that she is having trouble expressing herself well so she may speak less than she did before the TBI.

When the person with TBI cannot seem to find the right word when she needs it, she may get frustrated. She may express her frustration as irritability or even agitation. As a caregiver, you must understand the reason for her irritability. Reassure her and provide her a calm and soothing environment. Responding to her frustration with anger will likely agitate her even more and cause her to have more trouble expressing herself.

Encourage the person with TBI to put forth full effort in speech therapy. Being there for her during this intense therapy time, being patient with her as she relearns language skills, conversing with her and exposing her to language, can be very helpful.

Speech and Language Therapy

Treatment of language disorders caused by TBI primarily involves speech and language therapy. Many people with TBI improve their language substantially with aggressive therapy. Because in many cases people with TBI have more subtle language disorders than classic fluent or nonfluent aphasia, often anomia or aprosody, working with a speech and language pathologist well-versed in TBI is critical. Teasing apart how many of the person with TBI's cognitive problems are due to impairments in memory, how many are due to language impairments, and how many are due to altered mood may also require the expertise of a neuropsychiatric physician, neurologist, or psychiatrist familiar with TBI, working alongside a speech and language pathologist.

In the past, the dogma was that if language does not recover within six months, speech therapy should be discontinued. As we have learned more about the brain and its capacity for plasticity or adaptation, it has become clear that speech therapy is helpful for much longer than a few months after the injury. Although insurance coverage may be limited to a specific duration of time for therapy, longer and more extensive therapy is often useful in maximizing recovery. Practice at home, with family and friends, can be helpful as well.

Drug Therapy

There are limited data on whether medications help language dysfunction after TBI. Cognitive enhancers such as stimulants (like Ritalin [methylphenidate]) or acetylcholinesterase inhibitors (like Aricept [donepezil]) may help with cognition, but it is unclear whether they specifically help with language. These drugs may enhance cognition in general and improve language indirectly. Key elements to recovery are avoiding drugs and alcohol, maximizing social interaction, treating mood or anxiety problems, and engaging in speech therapy, with medication supplementation if needed.

In summary, language problems that develop after TBI often include issues with expression, trouble comprehending spoken language, difficulty with both expression and comprehension, and difficulty naming items. All these forms of language dysfunction may be associated with a loss of rhythm and melody in speech. Conversely, a person with TBI can lose melodic speech even though expression and comprehension are intact. The typical language problems after TBI tend to improve with speech therapy and the proper environment.

Tips for Coping with Language Problems after TBI

If you know someone who is experiencing language problems after TBI:

> Consult a speech-language therapist. A speech-language therapist can do many things to help your loved one with TBI who has language problems. A good speech-language therapist is the key to improving language difficulties after TBI.
>
> Attend the therapy sessions with the person experiencing language problems. Work with her at home as she practices the strategies she learns in therapy. During your practice sessions, ensure that the environment is calm and free from distractions. Try to make sure that the person with TBI is not tired and is able to pay attention and cooperate.

> Don't shout. Your loved one with TBI may have language problems, but she isn't deaf. Loud talk can upset or worsen her frustration.
> Keep communication simple, but do not treat an adult with brain injury like a child. Try to maintain as normal a life as possible by including her in family conversations.
> Seek professional help. If you notice symptoms such as dips in mood, tearfulness, or lack of interest in someone you are caring for, tell her doctor about these changes.

PART V

Other Common Problems Caused by the Traumatized Brain

We have explored the major emotional, behavioral, and cognitive symptoms seen after traumatic brain injury. In this part of the book, we discuss a few of the more common neurological symptoms that can occur after TBI: headaches, seizures, and vision problems. These symptoms can lead people with TBI to visit a neurologist at first, but there can be a psychiatric component to these conditions as well.

17

Headaches

Ashley was a sophomore in college and a star on the school's diving team. At practice one morning, she miscalculated as she attempted to execute a complex dive. She hit her head on the board and splashed into the pool below, unconscious. Her coach pulled her from the water as other team members called for an ambulance. Ashley woke up to paramedics strapping her to a life board and carrying her out of the pool house. In the ambulance, she felt confused and disoriented and vomited weakly during the short ride to the hospital. Emergency department staff took a CT scan of Ashley's head, and the results were normal. Doctors discharged Ashley that same day with the diagnosis of concussion.

Over the next two days, Ashley's confusion and tiredness improved, but she developed a severe headache. Her physician ordered another CT scan, and the results were again normal. Ashley continued to have headaches, which manifested in two forms: a dull pressure around her head, present most of the time, and worsening bouts of throbbing pain associated with vomiting and sensitivity to light. Her doctor advised her to get adequate rest, maintain a healthy lifestyle, and use Imitrex (sumatriptan) if necessary for her severe headaches. But the headaches persisted, and Ashley became frustrated and anxious. She wasn't sleeping, and she was falling behind at school. "My head hurts all the time," she said. At six months after her injury, seeing no improvement, Ashley's parents consulted a psychiatrist, who, after evaluating Ashley, prescribed Cymbalta (duloxetine) for the headache and anxiety symptoms and referred her to a therapist with expertise in mindfulness meditation. The combination of therapy and medications helped Ashley significantly, and she returned to school.

HEADACHES ARE A COMMON complaint after traumatic brain injury, particularly after mild TBI. Severe TBIs can also lead to headaches, vomiting, and severe pain, especially immediately after impact. If vomiting and severe pain occur after a TBI, seek medical attention immediately, because these symptoms can reflect increased pressure in the brain. Increased pressure in the brain is dangerous because the hard skull drastically limits where the brain can go when it is under pressure. In the worst cases, increased pressure shifts the brain and traps the brainstem—the part of the brain that connects to the spinal cord—in the back of the head, which can be fatal.

As times goes on, headaches can become a chronic problem. As we discuss in this chapter, there are many types of chronic headache, and many factors can influence how chronic the headaches become and what symptoms occur with them. Depression, anxiety, posttraumatic stress disorder, and sleep problems can all play a role and contribute to the chronic nature of the headaches and the intensity of the symptoms. Figure 17.1 depicts the complex relationship between TBI and post-TBI headaches and other factors that can prolong the headaches.

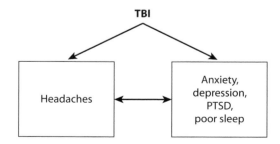

Figure 17.1. The complex interaction between TBI and headaches

Symptoms

Although headaches from a mild TBI are generally less severe than those from a severe TBI, they can nevertheless be persistent and problematic. They can be triggered or worsened by light and sound sensitivity, and they can be associated with dizziness. Most headaches resolve within the first few days to weeks and almost all within the first few months, but in some cases they do persist.

Table 17.1 lists common forms of chronic headache that develop after TBI. Tension-type headaches are common after TBI. These headaches often worsen as the day progresses. Tension-type headaches typically manifest as tightness in the neck and a feeling that there is a tight band around the head, but the sufferer has little or

TABLE 17.1 *Common Types of Chronic Headache after TBI*

Headache type	Characteristics
Tension	• Bilateral, dull pressure–like pain • Often triggered by stress
Migraine	• Often one-sided • Throbbing pain • May be associated with nausea, vomiting, or auras (for example, seeing flashes of light)
Occipital neuralgia	• Pain in the back of the head or on top of the head, in the neck, and behind the eyes; piercing • Pain worsens on neck movement • Can be associated with increased sensitivity to light
Cervicogenic	• Associated with neck pain and neck stiffness • May be one-sided or appear on both sides • Pain worsens in certain neck positions
Medication overuse	• Use of analgesics (ibuprofen, for example, for more than 15 days a month for more than 3 months)
Other causes	• Bleeding in the brain (sometimes indicated by a very severe headache, the worst in a lifetime). *Bleeding in the brain is a medical emergency.* If you suspect there is bleeding in the brain, call 911 immediately! • Brain surgery

no sensitivity to light or sound. These headaches often respond to Tylenol (acetaminophen) or Advil/Motrin (ibuprofen). In most cases, tension-type headaches do get better over time, but it may be worth consulting a headache specialist if these headaches persist for months. Nonmedication techniques such as massage and stress management can help alleviate tension-type headaches. It is also possible that overuse of medication is causing the headache: daily use of headache medications may, ironically, cause more headaches.

Headaches after TBI can mimic migraine headaches. Migraines often involve significant sensitivity to light and sound, and people with migraines report pulsing and pounding of the head. When these kinds of headache occur, the person suffering will likely want to be in a quiet, darkened room. Of course, what triggers a migraine varies from person to person, but common triggers include stress, lack of sleep, irregular sleep schedule (getting too much sleep on the weekend and too little sleep during the week), caffeine, and certain foods. Ashley, in our opening story, was experiencing a combination of tension-type and migraine headaches.

Treatment

There are multiple forms of treatment for post-TBI headache. For most people, headaches resolve on their own. In cases of chronic headache, medications can help; they are prescribed on the basis of type and cause of the headache. Stress management (with meditation and yoga), talk therapy (particularly cognitive behavioral therapy), exercise, adequate sleep, good nutrition, and support from family and friends are all important factors for alleviating post-TBI headache.

Drug Therapy

The two approaches to treating post-TBI migraines are either acute treatment for the current headaches only or regularly taking a medication to prevent or minimize future migraines. Acute treatment usually involves "triptan" medications such as Imitrex (sumatriptan), Zomig (zolmitriptan), or Relpax (eletriptan). Botox (botulinum toxin) injections can also be helpful for migraines, although Botox is usually reserved for people who have frequent migraines. For people who have frequent migraines, preventive therapy may also be beneficial. Preventive medications include Topamax (topiramate), Depakote (valproic acid), and Inderal (propranolol). Topamax may also help with impulsivity after TBI. Depakote, a mainstay of bipolar disorder treatment, may also help with irritability and agitation, which may develop after TBI. Incidentally, both Topamax and Depakote are antiseizure medications. Inderal is a medication for high blood pressure.

There is much overlap in the uses of these medications, so if the person with TBI is having multiple symptoms or medical problems, her physician may prescribe one medication to help treat several or all of them.

After TBI, it is also possible to have a mixed type of headache in which there is both a tension-type headache component and a migraine component, as Ashley experienced. These headache combinations can be challenging to treat, especially if they occur frequently months to years after the TBI. Mood problems like depression can complicate some people's response to medication. Depression and migraines (and possibly other types of headache) may make each other worse. There may also be some overlap in the neurophysiology and neurotransmitters involved. For example, medications that increase serotonin are mainstays of treatment for both depression and migraine (although they are different types of medication). Treatment of depression or anxiety may be a critical part of recovery from chronic headaches.

It is also possible that the post-TBI headache is not due to the TBI at all, or at least not *exclusively* to the TBI. Headaches are common throughout the general population and are not always the result of a TBI. The onset of headaches after TBI, especially chronic headaches, may be a coincidence. It could also be that the life changes and stresses associated with sustaining a brain injury might trigger headaches in someone who was already vulnerable to getting headaches (because of genetics, for example). Sometimes, headaches are accompanied by other symptoms, such as dizziness. Treating the dizziness directly may help, as dizziness can sometimes contribute to headache symptoms (dizziness in which the room appears to be spinning or things don't look stable in the environment can lead to headaches in some people).

In summary, headaches are not uncommon after TBI. Often, especially with chronic headaches, there are multiple factors involved. Mood problems, sleep disturbances, stress, and even certain medications can all affect whether someone has headaches after TBI and what kind of headaches she has.

Tips for Coping with Headaches after TBI

If you are experiencing headaches after TBI:

> If headaches are severe, chronic, persistent, or associated with vomiting or blurred vision, contact your primary care doctor.

> Maintain a healthy lifestyle. Despite the headache, try to get some form of regular exercise. Keep a structured daily routine, stay engaged with hobbies, practice good sleep hygiene (see Chapter 12), and take steps to manage your stress.

> Find your stress buster. Find out what relaxes you and do it! Meditation techniques such as mindfulness, repeating a mantra (a word or a phrase), or tensing and relaxing parts of your body can help with relaxation. Rhythmic breathing or yoga techniques can help as well.

> Find your headache triggers and avoid them. Triggers can come in many forms, including dietary components, stressful situations, or excessive stimulation. Triggers can include certain foods (such as chocolate) or lack of certain foods (coffee, if you normally have something caffeinated every day). Too little or even too much sleep can trigger headaches.

> Do not overuse pain medications. Excessive use of pain medications can make headaches worse.

> If you have mood, anxiety, or other emotional symptoms, consult a psychiatrist or therapist. These professionals can make appropriate referrals if you need more or different approaches to headache treatment than they have to offer.

18

Seizures

Rashad, a 33-year-old architect, sustained a severe traumatic brain injury when three men assaulted him in the alley behind his office. The men surrounded Rashad and demanded his wallet. When he refused, they beat him, kicked him repeatedly in the head and neck, then robbed him and left him sprawled in the alley. A passerby, who found him bleeding from his nose, with fluid draining from his ears, called 911 for help. An ambulance rushed Rashad to the emergency department. By this time, Rashad was comatose. Examination showed he had multiple contusions and bleeding inside his brain. Rashad was admitted to the Neurocritical Care Unit and underwent brain surgery to remove a blood clot. He received antiseizure medication for seven days. After two weeks in the Neurocritical Care Unit, he was transferred to an inpatient rehabilitation facility, where he continued to make good progress. He was discharged five weeks after the assault.

Rashad continued to do well after returning home, but about six months after the injury, he began to have seizures. "I black out. I black out *a lot*," he said. A neurologist evaluated Rashad, diagnosed him with secondarily generalized seizures, and started him on antiseizure medications.

SEIZURES CAN OCCUR IMMEDIATELY after a TBI (within the first 24 hours), early (within the first week), or late (beyond the first week). Late seizures have the highest risk of leading to an ongoing seizure disorder, called epilepsy. Seizures are often associated with mood, cognitive, or behavioral problems, and they can complicate recovery from TBI.

What Is a Seizure?

Seizures, or convulsions, happen when the brain's electrical system malfunctions. Normally, the brain discharges electrical energy in an organized, controlled manner that permits the brain cells to communicate with one another. But when the brain's electrical system malfunctions, the brain cells fire in a disorganized manner and keep on firing. The resulting surge of energy through the brain can cause loss of consciousness and muscle contractions.

Seizures can last anywhere from a few seconds to a couple of minutes, but the person can be confused after a seizure, and this postseizure confusion can last for minutes or as long as several hours. A seizure that persists for several minutes is a medical emergency requiring immediate hospitalization. The word *epilepsy* refers to a disorder in which a person experiences more than two unprovoked seizures.

The two broad categories of seizure are partial seizures and generalized seizures. Partial seizures affect only part of the brain. Generalized seizures act diffusely and affect the entire brain. The phrase *secondarily generalized seizure* describes a partial seizure that spreads and becomes generalized. This form of seizure is common after a TBI. Rashad, in our opening story, developed secondarily generalized seizures.

Generalized Seizures

The classic image of seizure—someone getting stiff and shaking—is in fact a type of generalized seizure called a tonic-clonic seizure, or grand mal seizure. In this kind of seizure, the person loses consciousness and may bite his tongue or lose control of his bladder. The person is usually tired and confused after the seizure. Tonic-clonic seizures can be scary to witness, but they are even more dangerous to the person having the seizure. If your loved one is having a tonic-clonic seizure for the first time, or if the person has had seizures before but the seizure duration is unusually long, call 911. A tonic-clonic seizure that lasts more than a few minutes increases the risk of cutting·off oxygen to the brain and subsequent brain damage.

Partial Seizures

A partial seizure is less obvious than a generalized tonic-clonic seizure. Partial seizures are subdivided into simple partial seizures, in which the person does not lose awareness or become confused, and complex partial seizures, in which either the person loses awareness or becomes confused during the time of the seizure.

The manifestations of a partial seizure vary by the location in the brain. If the seizure is in the frontal lobe, the person can feel that someone or something is forcing thoughts or actions on him. Temporal lobe seizures create a sense of fear, déjà vu (the feeling that one has already seen or experienced something), a rising sensation from the abdomen (like the feeling on a roller coaster), and even hallucinations and the sense that things are not real. Temporal lobe seizures can lead to vertigo or trouble with speech. Parietal lobe seizures can lead to odd body sensations. Occipital lobe seizures can lead to visual hallucinations. As you can see, partial seizures can be difficult to recognize.

A person having a partial seizure can experience mood changes (sadness, anger, fear), cognitive changes (feeling as if they are in a dream, mystical experiences, memory problems), or psychotic symptoms (such as hallucinations) before, during, or after the seizure.

If any one of these changes occurs at the time of the seizure, it can be hard to determine whether the symptoms indicate a seizure. A key factor to consider is how long the symptoms last. Seizures can last seconds to a few minutes. Another factor is that seizures are stereotyped to each person, which means that the symptoms appear essentially the same in that person for each seizure.

Partial seizures can induce a panicky sensation, which can be hard to differentiate from a panic attack. Again, remember that seizures last seconds to minutes, whereas panic attacks tend to last longer. Seizures occur suddenly, often without warning. Panic attacks may build up over time and can be brought on by a stressor or trigger (such as being in enclosed spaces for those who have claustrophobia). The panic or fear from a seizure, on the other hand, does not build up; it occurs at a maximum level immediately.

Seizures can cause other anxiety symptoms that are easily confused with anxiety disorders. A person having a seizure may feel that the world around him is not real (derealization) or that he himself is not real (depersonalization). Such surreal experiences can lead to anxiety. Partial seizures originating in the temporal lobe can cause these sensations; partial seizures affecting the amygdala (deep within the brain near the temporal lobe) can lead to panic.

Besides panic and anxiety, partial seizures that affect the temporal lobe can lead to cognitive issues, like memory impairment or déjà vu, or to psychotic symptoms.

Traumatic brain injury can also cause complex partial seizure episodes that in some way impair the person's consciousness. The person may be confused or completely unaware of his surroundings during such seizures. Complex partial seizures often can originate in the temporal and frontal lobes, and given that these areas are particularly vulnerable to injury, such seizures may occur after TBI.

Why do some people have seizures after traumatic brain injury and others do not? The answer may lie in part with the severity of the TBI. The more severe the TBI, the more likely it is, in general, that seizures will develop. Bleeding in the brain increases the risk of seizures, partly because blood irritates the brain. Penetrating brain injuries (in which an object penetrates the scalp and brain) are more likely to lead to seizures than are closed head injuries (in which there is no penetration). Increased age and a family history of epilepsy also increase the risk of developing seizures after a TBI.

Having a seizure within the first 24 hours to a week after the TBI does not mean that the person will necessarily develop epilepsy. These early seizures can be a result of physical and metabolic changes in the brain that occurred soon after the injury. Late seizures can be related to structural changes and scarring in the brain.

Epilepsy

Our discussion thus far has focused on the acute issues related to seizures after TBI. But the person with TBI who develops epilepsy faces a different set of challenges. For example, people with TBI who have epilepsy have an increased risk of developing mood and anxiety problems. Depression can be common in epilepsy and may even be a greater influence on quality of life than the type or frequency of the seizures. Luckily, depression with epilepsy responds to typically used antidepressants. Treating the depression not only improves quality of life but may also impact the seizures themselves.

People with TBI who develop epilepsy may also be vulnerable to symptoms like hallucinations or delusions as part of the seizure, right after a seizure, or as an ongoing problem between seizures. Treatment with antipsychotics is necessary for some of these people, particularly when psychotic symptoms continue between seizures. If the psychotic symptoms occur during or after seizures, the best treatment may be antiseizure medications.

Nonepileptic Seizures

Some people with TBI develop nonepileptic seizures (NES). Non-epileptic seizures are spells that are not detectable with standard diagnostic tests, such as an electroencephalogram (EEG), and they are unusual in their presentation in some ways. For example, a person experiencing a NES may thrash around, but his arms and legs are not coordinated together as typically happens in epileptic seizures, or he may be moving all parts of his body but be able to respond at the same time. NES is considered a conversion disorder. We don't understand conversion disorder very well, but we do know that in some people, "psychological" symptoms "convert" to neurological symptoms such as seizures. Conversion is not malingering; that is, the person who has these symptoms is not knowingly making them up. Rather, we believe subconscious mental stress or distress generates these symptoms. Nonepileptic seizures are best treated by working with a psychiatrist, a psychologist, or a therapist.

It can be difficult even for experts to distinguish nonepileptic seizures from epilepsy. To complicate this further, some people with epileptic seizures can also experience NES. Also, an EEG may not detect the source if the seizure originated deep within the brain. EEG electrodes are placed on the scalp, so the seizures they capture best are those near the scalp as opposed to deep within the brain. The type of EEG may be a factor in picking up a seizure: a regular EEG is not as sensitive in picking up seizures as an ambulatory EEG, which records electrical activity over 24 or 48 hours. Even more effective is monitoring for 48 or 72 hours in an inpatient epilepsy monitoring unit. Even under these conditions, however, technicians may miss a deep seizure. Finally, a seizure disorder cannot always be ruled out even if the patient shows no clinical symptoms (and hence no EEG abnormalities) during monitoring.

Treatment

People who have early seizures are often treated with antiseizure medications for about a week to prevent further seizures and brain damage from lack of oxygen. Even patients who have not had seizures but appear to be at risk are treated with antiseizure medications for about a week. Rashad did not have an early seizure, but because he had a severe injury, his doctors considered him to be "at risk" and prescribed antiseizure medication.

People who have late-onset seizures receive medication after the seizures begin. The neurologist determines when to start and stop antiseizure medications and what type of medicine to use. The onset of late seizures is unpredictable; evidence shows an elevated risk for a first seizure 10 or even 20 years after severe brain injury.

Antiepileptic medications can have mood, behavioral, and cognitive side effects. Certain antiepileptics, like Topamax (topiramate) and Dilantin (phenytoin), can cause cognitive side effects (problems with memory or finding the right word when needed). Keppra (levetiracetam) can lead to irritability, agitation, and depression in some patients. On the other hand, if the person with TBI has trouble with mood stability, some antiepileptic medications, such as Lamictal (lamotrigine), Depakote (valproic acid), or Tegretol (carbamazepine), may be helpful with mood as well as seizure control. Lyrica (prega-balin) or Neurontin (gabapentin) may help the person with TBI who has anxiety problems. Another thing to be aware of is drug-drug interactions between antiepileptics and other medications the person with TBI is taking, because such interactions can affect both the person's tolerance and the effectiveness of the antiepileptic.

In summary, seizures can occur after TBI and are more common in moderate and severe TBI than in mild TBI. Seizures can manifest in many different ways: they can be partial or generalized or start partially and become generalized. In addition, seizures can occur with or without loss of consciousness. Emotional and behavioral problems are common in people with seizures.

If you or the person you are caring for has had seizures after TBI, seek professional help from a neurologist and follow his or her recommendations. Having a seizure or seizures after TBI is no guarantee that epilepsy (that is, recurrent seizures) will develop. On the other hand, there can be an increased risk of seizures years after the TBI. The good news is that there are a number of medications to treat seizures, and chances are good that these medications will control the seizures.

Tips for Coping with Seizures after TBI

If you know someone who is experiencing seizures after TBI:

> Safety comes first and trumps all other issues: Keep the person having a seizure safe. If he is seated and having a seizure, hold him to make sure he does not fall. If he is standing, gently lower him to the floor. Turn him onto his left side to prevent him from aspirating saliva into the lungs. Loosen any tight clothes around his neck. Do not put anything in his mouth.

Call 911 if:

- this is the first time the person is having a seizure,
- the seizure lasts longer than three to five minutes, or
- the person does not resume normal breathing after the seizure ends.

If the person has had seizures before or if the seizure lasts less than several minutes, inform his doctor about the episode.

> Use the buddy system for high-risk activities: People who have post-TBI seizures should never be alone when performing activities such as bathing, swimming, climbing heights, or operating machines.
> Learn your state's regulations on driving. A person with post-TBI seizures should consult his neurologist and follow his or her recommendations about when it is safe to drive again. States' regulations vary regarding how long someone must be seizure-free before a person with seizures is allowed to drive.
> If you notice mood, cognitive, or behavioral symptoms in your loved one with TBI and seizures, encourage him to consult his doctor. He may need additional treatment from a psychiatrist or a therapist.
> Be alert to specific triggers that provoke seizures. Common triggers include bright lights, alcohol or illicit drug use, alcohol withdrawal, and irregular sleep patterns. For people who are prescribed antiseizure medication, the most common trigger for seizure is *not* taking the medication.

19

Vision

Staff Sergeant Patrice's third tour of duty in Afghanistan ended with an explosion. She and her unit hit an IED as they rode cautiously through a deserted town. The explosion slammed Patrice, who was riding inside the tank, up against the roof. She and the other surviving soldiers radioed for help and were airlifted back to base, where medical personnel diagnosed Patrice with a broken left arm and a moderate traumatic brain injury. Within two days, 30-year-old Patrice was recovering at an army medical center back in the United States.

Although Patrice's arm healed quickly, her brain injury led to several physical problems, including difficulties with walking, balance, speech, and vision. Her visual problems included increased sensitivity to light, blurred vision, and, periodically, double vision. The examining physician noted that Patrice had difficulty moving her eyes in all directions. These visual problems were very troubling to Patrice, and she wondered if she would ever be able to do what she could do before. "I'm seeing double so much of the time now," she said. "I'm always knocking my coffee cup over."

TBI CAN LEAD to a range of vision problems, including double vision, trouble keeping the eyes in place while reading (maintaining focus), blurred vision, sensitivity to light, eye strain, depth perception dysfunction, and inability to see part of the environment. Chronic visual problems are more common in moderate to severe TBI than in mild TBI, though people can have problems with their vision (like double or blurry vision) for a few days to weeks after a mild TBI. Diagnosing and treating visual problems in TBI is particularly important because any visual disturbance, no matter how slight, can impede a person's ability to fully participate in and improve with physical therapy after TBI. Furthermore, because vision is a critical sense for us, visual problems can be very disconcerting to people, and they contribute to depression and anxiety problems.

The specific visual problem that occurs after TBI depends on both the severity of the TBI and the location of the damage. Visual problems can originate in the eye itself, in the optic nerve (which connects the eyes to the brain), or in any of the multiple regions in the brain that transmit and process visual information.

How TBI Affects Vision

Traumatic brain injury can directly damage the eyes and the optic nerves. In a car accident, for example, the impact can propel the driver through the windshield, directly traumatizing the face and eyes. People with damage to the retinas, the layer of cells in the back of the eyeball, may see floaters (or floating spots), or even small pieces of tissue floating within the eyeball. Direct or indirect injury to the optic nerves (called traumatic optic neuropathy) is one of the most serious visual problems that can result from TBI.

TBI can damage the visual pathways connecting the cell groupings in the brain that process visual information. Because each of these cell groupings carries out different functions, damage to them leads to different visual symptoms. To explain this in greater detail, we'll next discuss the brain's visual pathways, then explore where and how these pathways can sustain damage.

When we look out at the world, we usually assume that our brain is faithfully reproducing the world out there. In truth, however, what we see is an illusion. Instead, the brain builds a model of visual reality out of information that it receives through the eyes. The world "out there" is composed of light that oscillates at different frequencies, some of which we can see and some of which we cannot (ultraviolet and infrared light are two examples of light we cannot see). The brain quickly, efficiently, and automatically converts these light waves into a model of the world that we recognize and assume is there.

This concept may seem radical, but neuroscience leaves no doubt that the brain alone is the architect of the world we see. To illustrate this, consider that our eyes continuously move slightly, even when we are still. Our eyes are moving as we walk, too. But as we walk, we don't see the world as blurred moving images, do we? Instead, we see the world as a stable backdrop because the brain is continually making adjustments to how it perceives the world. In addition, our eyes project information from the world to our brains upside down! Our brain inverts the image, so that we don't even know that the information we had originally was upside down!

At a deeper level, different parts of the brain receive information describing the color, shape, and movement of an object. The brain has to blend or bind all this information together so that when we look out at the world, we see all aspects of the object simultaneously—that is, we see the color, shape, and other attributes of the object instantly and at the same location in space. The brain combines this information and other information instantaneously, so we don't even know that it is happening or appreciate the amount of work that goes into it.

TBI can disrupt the extensive brain circuitry that carries out these amazing feats. Vision circuitry involves pathways that lead from the retinas to an area called the optic chiasm, and then to the lateral geniculate nucleus of the thalamus. This area of the thalamus relays visual information to the occipital cortex (the primary visual center) and to the superior colliculus, in the midbrain, which directs eye movements.

Axons (nerve cell fibers) in the retina at the back of the eye exit the retina bundled together as the optic nerve. At the optic chiasm, a partial joining of information from the two eyes joins the fibers from each eye that receive input from the same area in space. Information reaches the lateral geniculate nucleus of the thalamus on each side and is then relayed to the occipital lobe of each hemisphere of the brain. The left occipital cortex receives information about the right side of the world from both eyes, and the right occipital cortex receives information about the left side of the world from both eyes.

From the occipital cortex, information can travel via either the ventral pathway (the "what" pathway) or the dorsal pathway (the "where" pathway). The ventral pathway passes through the inferior temporal lobe and is associated with recognizing objects ("what" things are). The dorsal pathway passes through the middle temporal lobe to the parietal lobe and is associated with motion and spatial vision ("where" things are).

Where in these circuits the damage occurred determines what specific visual problem a person with TBI has. Damage to the optic nerve from one eye can lead to complete visual loss from that eye. Damage at the optic chiasm can lead to lack of vision from parts of both eyes. People can also have "holes" in their vision (called scotomas), spots in the visual field where vision is absent or deficient.

Severe TBI can damage the optic chiasm; severe TBI can also affect the fibers that run from the optic chiasm to the thalamus and then to the occipital lobe, causing blindness in part of the visual field from both eyes (called visual field cuts), or scotomas. Damage to the fibers on the right side of the brain can lead to loss of vision on the left visual field and vice versa. Damage to the occipital lobes can lead to total blindness. In a condition called Anton's syndrome, people with damage to the occipital lobes are not able to see, but do not accept that they are blind and confabulate a visual image. Sadly, their brains are unable to recognize that they are blind; they are not lying or making up things to deceive you.

In addition to the fibers connecting the eyes to the occipital lobes are fibers that connect the eyes to specific regions of the brainstem. These areas control eye movements, so damage to these regions can lead to blurry or double vision, the very problems that Patrice complained of in our opening story. Although this condition is more common in cases of moderate and severe TBI, it is not uncommon in mild TBI.

Three cranial nerves, numbers III, IV, and VI, are located in the middle of the brainstem. These nerves control the eye movements and can be damaged by injury to the back of the brain, where the brainstem is. Damage to these pathways can impair the ability of both eyes to focus on the same spot, leading to eye strain and blurry vision, or cause uncoordinated movements of the eyes, creating double vision. Severe TBI can misalign one or both eyes. Comprehensive eye examination revealed that Patrice had damage to the nerves responsible for moving the eyes.

Rarely, visual problems can develop from impaired perception of one's surroundings, due to damage to the dorsal visual pathway that leads to the parietal lobe. People who suffer this injury completely neglect one "side" of space and are aware of and act in only one side of space. A man would shave only one side of his face, for example, or a woman would apply makeup to only one eye or put clothes on only one side of her body, simply because they are not aware of the other side of space. This phenomenon (called unilateral spatial neglect) is more common after a stroke, but it can occur with TBI.

Light sensitivity can also develop after TBI. The person with TBI may feel pain or discomfort in her eyes when she is exposed to light. We're not sure why this occurs, although one hypothesis is that it is associated with changes in blood flow in the brain after brain injury.

Treatment

The mainstay of treatment for visual problems after TBI is visual rehabilitation, a process of educating and training people with visual deficits to achieve maximum visual function and optimal quality of life. Eye physicians (ophthalmologists), optometrists, or a team of specially trained professionals can provide visual rehabilitation. A visual therapist tailors the specific rehabilitation strategy to the source of the problem—the eyes, the optic nerves, the visual areas of the brain, or the cranial nerves in the brainstem.

Surgery may be necessary if the retina is damaged or detached from the tissue around it. If the person with TBI experiences blurred vision and the problem appears to originate in the eyes themselves, then prescription eyeglasses or contact lenses may be appropriate.

Refractive prisms may be used in rehabilitation to help the blurriness improve.

If there is damage to the optic nerve, steroids may be used soon after the brain damage; surgery may also be necessary in the early stages of injury. Damage to the visual pathways may require surgery to remove blood from the brain or a temporary course of steroids. Unfortunately, TBI can lead to permanent visual problems because the damage may be subtle or may not be responsive to medical or surgical treatment. In these cases, visual rehabilitation can teach strategies that compensate for lost or diminished vision. Special tinted lenses that decrease light sensitivity, or prism lenses or eye patches to treat double vision, may be helpful.

Because vision is a critical sense to most people, visual problems can lead to anxiety and depressive symptoms. It is important to address these symptoms and treat them, as the mood and anxiety symptoms can affect rehabilitation and make recovery more difficult. This can become a circular problem, as poor rehabilitation can lead to no improvement of symptoms, which can lead to worsening anxiety or depression.

In summary, visual problems can and do occur after traumatic brain injury. Because vision is one of the critical senses and because we rely heavily on visual information to navigate the world, restoring vision quickly is a priority in those who suffer a TBI. Addressing vision problems as quickly as possible after TBI maximizes the person's benefit from overall rehabilitation because she is better able to follow therapy instructions. Depression or anxiety symptoms after visual problems should be treated aggressively.

Tips for Coping with Visual Problems after TBI
If you are experiencing visual problems after TBI:

> Consult an eye specialist (ophthalmologist or optometrist) if you are concerned about your vision. An eye specialist may refer you to a neuro-ophthalmologist (a superspecialist with expertise in brain injury) or to a visual rehabilitation therapist or both.

If you know someone who is experiencing visual problems after TBI:

> Reduce clutter and keep the home organized. Simple and powerful tools to help the person with TBI and visual problems include having clear walking pathways, organized work spaces, and cueing systems to help your loved one identify objects or locations (one example is attaching a guide string leading from the kitchen table to the bathroom).

> Offer emotional support. Having visual problems after a TBI can be a very frightening experience. It is often only after an injury affects our vision that it becomes clear how dependent we really are on this sense. One of the best things you can do for the person with brain injury who is having visual deficits is to offer your emotional support.

Epilogue

Leslie is a 41-year-old school teacher, a wife, and the mother of two young children. Her car collided with another car as she pulled out of the school parking lot one afternoon. Leslie was sober and wearing her seatbelt when she was hit. Paramedics found her unconscious at the scene of the accident, but she gradually regained consciousness by the time the ambulance arrived at the emergency department. A CT scan revealed contusions in the left side of the brain and a small bleed outside the brain (subdural hematoma), also on the left side. Leslie had sustained a moderately severe traumatic brain injury. The doctors opted not to do brain surgery. But Leslie developed weakness on the right side and had difficulty using her right hand and right leg.

Leslie received physical therapy (PT) in the hospital. Her doctors discharged her about two weeks after the accident, recommending that she receive outpatient physical therapy and that a neurologist and her primary care doctor monitor her progress.

Leslie continued with PT after her discharge but progressed slowly. Over the next few weeks, she also developed intermittent headaches, poor sleep, and fatigue, and she could not keep up with her responsibilities at the school. Leslie eventually had to take a leave of absence. She saw her doctors regularly and received treatment with various medicines for the headaches and insomnia. She returned to work three months after the accident, but even then she felt that she wasn't efficient. She still wasn't driving, and she dragged her right leg a little—though her arm felt much better now.

As months went by, Leslie's husband noticed that she was sad, tearful, easily frustrated, and quiet. She was not spending time with the family; she came home from work tired and went straight to bed. About nine months after the accident, Leslie admitted to her husband that she just couldn't take it anymore; she needed professional help.

Together they consulted with their primary care doctor, who diagnosed Leslie with clinical depression and referred her to a neuropsychiatrist. The neuropsychiatrist confirmed the clinical depression diagnosis and saw Leslie regularly. He tried several different medications before he found a medicine that worked for Leslie. Meanwhile, he recommended that she maintain a timetable for the day, go to sleep and wake up around the same time every day, exercise for at least 20 minutes every day, and eat a healthy diet. He recommended some booster sessions of physical therapy to help her regain her strength, a few sessions of occupational therapy, and weekly sessions with a mental health therapist.

It took some time for Leslie's symptoms to improve, but after three months she was doing much better. She felt better, she looked better, she had energy, and she found renewed inspiration for teaching her students.

WE HAVE HAD a long journey together over the course of this book, exploring the structure and function of the brain, the various ways traumatic brain injury affects the brain, and the emotional, behavioral, cognitive, and general neurological symptoms of the traumatized brain.

In this chapter, we synthesize what we have discussed throughout the book and summarize our recommendations. Our ultimate goal is to help you or the person you are caring for learn how to recover from the trauma of brain injury.

Leslie, in our opening story, is a patient of ours who sustained a moderately severe TBI and developed depression after her injury.

Her positive attitude, her compliance with the treatment plan, and the support of her family were all keys to her recovery. Her depressive symptoms resolved in a few months, and she was able to get back to her previous level of functioning. Everything that Leslie did is doable. We present her story to show that neuropsychiatric symptoms after TBI are indeed treatable. Do not ignore them or be ashamed of them. Get help.

Leslie's story epitomizes what can be done to optimize outcomes in brain injury. Most importantly, Leslie was willing to accept what happened and do everything she could to recover. There is a trauma—a psychological trauma—when a sudden event occurs that upends our lives. Dealing with this trauma and accepting what happened is an important part of recovery for the traumatized brain.

Let's explore some of the specific reasons why Leslie's recovery went so well in the end. These are simple steps and techniques that you or your loved one with brain injury can also implement to help in recovery from TBI.

Medical Records. Leslie brought all her medical records, including records of her hospitalization, to her first appointment with the neuropsychiatrist. Her records helped the doctor get a good understanding of Leslie's injury without having to speculate about what exactly happened in the accident and how severe her brain injury was. Having this information is valuable to a doctor because many patients with brain injury do not remember the sequence of events right before, during, or after the injury. Having a record of Leslie's medical history and previous medications helped the doctor choose a medication that Leslie had not tried. Without these records, the doctor may have prescribed a medication that Leslie had tried before and that didn't help her, leading to inefficient care and further delays in her recovery.

> ❯ What you can do: Arrange for the doctors who are treating the person with TBI to receive copies of all the person's medical records from the accident, as well as her full medical history, including all current and previous medications.

Medical Advocate or Companion. Leslie's husband accompanied her to most of her medical appointments. He was able to give a lot more information about Leslie's mood state and how it was impacting her, information that gave the doctor a better perspective on Leslie's illness. Because of the nature of mood, behavioral, and cognitive symptoms, the person with TBI may have little insight into her symptoms.

> What you can do: Be sure that a responsible adult accompanies the person with TBI to most if not all medical appointments, if possible. The medical advocate can take notes, answer questions that the person with TBI may not be able to answer, and be aware of the doctor's recommendations for treatment.

Medication and Therapy Compliance. Leslie's compliance and willingness to follow recommendations served her well. She carefully followed the occupational therapist's recommendations for structuring her day and gradually building in new activities. She attended the physical therapy sessions and regularly practiced her PT exercises at home. She met weekly with the psychotherapist and used the sessions to grieve, discuss her losses, and accept her new deficit—the mild right-sided weakness. She also learned the importance of continuing to take her medications to keep her moods in balance.

> What you can do: Work with the person with TBI to find ways to keep her on track with treatment therapies and taking medications as prescribed. Enter all appointments on a calendar or day-tracker that the person can refer to daily. Leave notes or reminders or set alarms to remind the person when to take medications.

The above practices will serve anyone well. We provided "Tips" in Chapters 5–19 to help with specific conditions. Here we offer some general guidelines for recovery from a traumatic brain injury.

General Guidelines for Recovery from a TBI

If you are a caregiver or family member of a person who is recovering from a traumatic brain injury:

> Be supportive.
> Educate yourself about TBI. Read, talk to professionals, or participate in a brain injury support group. Brain injury

support groups are a great venue for interacting with other people with TBI and caregivers and families involved in the care of people with TBI.

> Encourage the person you are caring for to seek professional help if you see that he or she is developing emotional, cognitive, or behavioral problems after a TBI.

> Safety first. If the person with TBI shows or experiences a sudden change in mood, behavior, or cognition, or if the person becomes violent or aggressive, seek immediate professional help. Call 911 or emergency medical services if you believe anyone is in danger.

> Work with the person with TBI to ensure that he or she is taking medications as prescribed and following all physicians' and therapists' recommendations. This can be a challenging task, but things will improve as you continue to closely work with the person who has suffered a TBI. There is no formula or recipe for how to do this; you can find support and encouragement in working with someone who has expertise in this area (doctor, therapist) or interacting with someone who has similar experiences with TBI (for example, attending brain injury support groups, discussing your issues, and getting feedback).

> Be creative; think outside the box. TBI injuries come in all shapes and sizes, and so do people. Don't be afraid to be unconventional in how you or the person with brain injury tackle challenges. (One of our patients pinned a note to her shirt, upside-down, so that she could look down and read it; that way she remembered to buy dog food at the supermarket on her way home from a physical therapy appointment.)

> Reward or praise the person with TBI when they do positive things and be sincere in your praise.

> Take care of yourself. Take breaks when you get tired or frustrated. You can't motivate the person with TBI if you yourself are run down and feeling discouraged.

> Don't hesitate to ask for help if you are constantly feeling burdened and down. If you are having difficulties with your spouse or other family members, consider marital or family

counseling. If you need a break, ask a trusted neighbor, friend, or family member to step in for a day or an afternoon.

If you are recovering from a traumatic brain injury:

> Educate yourself about TBI. Start by talking to your doctor. Ask questions about the severity of your injury, the likely course it may take, and do's and don'ts.
> Protect yourself against a second injury. Take simple precautions, such as wearing a helmet when biking, wearing a seatbelt, and not driving under the influence of alcohol.
> It is best that you abstain from drinking alcohol or using illicit drugs. Even though marijuana may be legal in some states, the marijuana available on the streets is not for your use, as you cannot know what other ingredients it contains. Labeling the percentage of the active ingredient is also not always accurate and consistent.
> Remember that working with a professional can help you gain a better understanding of your unique situation and teach you strategies to deal with your challenges. There is no reason to feel ashamed or embarrassed about getting help for these problems.

Hope for the Future

We want to share some promising future directions in the care of TBI.

Biomarkers

One of the difficulties in accurately diagnosing and treating those with traumatic brain injury is that sometimes there is not a good way to see the damage to the brain, especially if it is mild, on brain scans like CT scans. It would be very beneficial if there were biomarkers that correlate with brain injury and perhaps with recovery from the injury, just like there are blood tests that are done, for example, to detect poor thyroid functioning and monitor recovery from the illness. Luckily, there may be such markers of brain injury. Although still in the research stage as of this writing, some candidates look promising. In particular, BDNF (Brain Derived Neurotrophic Factor) levels may indicate severity of traumatic brain injury and, perhaps more importantly, track recovery from TBI. BDNF may also be an important marker for recovery from major depression, which suggests that the "neurological" and the "psychiatric" often overlap when we are talking about the brain. In addition to BDNF, researchers are also looking at other protein, lipid, inflammatory, and brain imaging markers. We are optimistic that we may in the future use markers to diagnose concussions (mild brain injuries) and predict who is likely to have bad consequences after brain injury.

Pharmacogenetic Testing

In pharmacogenetic testing the doctor swabs the inside of the cheek and sends the cells off for genetic testing. The tests reveal what genetic variants are in those cells that may affect the person's response to medications. For example, a person may have two versions of the "long" allele of the serotonin transporter, which might suggest that he or she is a good candidate for treatment with selective serotonin reuptake inhibitor (SSRI) medications. Pharmacogenetic testing also helps physicians determine which medications might work better based on how and how well a person metabolizes different medications. Pharmacogenetic testing has the potential to help with medication dosing and knowing which medications may be more likely to cause side effects. The indications, risks, and benefits of pharmacogenetic testing are still being worked out, but some physicians are currently using this testing.

Neuromodulation Techniques

One of the most exciting developments is the use of nonmedication interventions that directly impact the circuitry of the brain. Transcranial magnetic stimulation (TMS) is one such intervention. In TMS, a repeated magnetic pulse is used to slowly, over several weeks, change the electrical properties of certain circuits in the brain. The US Food and Drug Administration has approved TMS for treating major depression in the general population, and TMS is clinically available for this use. Because of its success in the general population, there is much research interest in using TMS for TBI.

Two other neuromodulation techniques in development and under investigation are transient direct current stimulation and deep brain stimulation. Transient direct current stimulation uses a mild electrical current to stimulate parts of the brain. Deep brain stimulation uses electrodes surgically implanted in selected areas of the brain to improve functioning.

These exciting developments are all still in the research stage. But, now that we have learned more and more about the pathways of the brain and how mood, behavioral, and cognitive symptoms occur when these pathways are interrupted or damaged, we are reaching the point where it may be possible to manipulate brain pathways to improve symptoms.

All these research advances have great implications for those who develop psychiatric symptoms after TBI. It is all the more important now that you or your loved one with TBI realize what these symptoms are and not be ashamed to get help. As you have learned by reading this book, these symptoms are real; they are not "made up." Doctors and research experts in brain injury now appreciate more than ever the importance of treating emotional, behavioral, and cognitive symptoms that develop after a TBI. Our knowledge and understanding of the neuroanatomy and treatment of brain injury is fast improving. Brain injury experts appreciate more than ever that emotional, behavioral, and cognitive symptoms can be related to the trauma just as much as such physical symptoms like weakness or loss of sensation.

Our aim in this book is to help those with TBI and their family members and caregivers understand their symptoms and how to improve them. We also want to teach people that psychiatric symptoms are real and are directly related to brain injury. There should be no shame, no suffering in silence. We are at the beginning of a landmark period in how we think about psychiatric symptoms; we are nearing the time when we can erase completely any lingering stigma still associated with psychiatry and mental illness. With this understanding, along with some support and hard work from family members and caregivers, persons with brain injury will recover optimally, in every sense of that word, from a traumatized brain.

GLOSSARY

aggression. Hostile, harmful, or destructive behavior that can be physical or verbal and can range from irritability to physical assault on others.

anomia. Difficulty in naming objects.

anxiety. An overwhelming sense of apprehension or fear.

apathy. A decrease in or lack of motivation.

aphasia. Disturbance of expression and comprehension of spoken language.

aprosody. Difficulty in appreciating or portraying emotions in speech.

arousal. The state of wakefulness that allows us to interact with the environment.

attention. Selection of one stimulus from the environment.

axon. A branch that extends from the soma, or body of the brain cell. Axons transmit signals to other neurons.

blast injury. Injury that results from exposure to an explosion, often encountered in the context of war or combat. Shock waves from the explosion damage the brain because of the sudden change in pressure brought on by the exploding device.

chronic traumatic encephalopathy (CTE). The developing concept that accumulated damage from a series of mild TBIs may lead to long-term impairment over the years.

circadian rhythm disorder. Disorders of the timing of sleep; for example, going to bed very early or very late or arising very early or very late.

clinical depression. A medical diagnosis describing sustained, persistent low (depressed) mood in a person who may not enjoy usual activities and who may have physical symptoms in addition to depressed mood, leading to impairment in day-to-day functioning.

cognitive behavioral therapy (CBT). A form of psychotherapy that is based on the principle that thoughts influence a person's feelings and behavior. CBT trains the patient to think more like a scientist, to examine whether the thoughts they are having are valid or supported by evidence.

complex partial seizure. A seizure in which the person has an alteration of awareness, but does not have stiffening and rhythmic movements.

computerized tomography scan (CT scan). An imaging technique that produces computer processed X-ray images of cross-sections of the body.

contusion. Bruising of the brain.

coup-contrecoup injury. A common pattern of head injury in which brain damage occurs both at the site of impact (the coup injury) and on the opposite side of the head from the impact (the contrecoup injury).

delusions. Firm, fixed, false beliefs that a person has, despite evidence to the contrary.

dendrite. A branch that extends from the soma. Dendrites receive signals from other neurons.

dialectical behavioral therapy (DBT). A form of psychotherapy that focuses on distressing problematic behaviors and helps the patient learn different, more rewarding approaches.

diffuse axonal injury (DAI). Damage to the axons as they are stretched in the back-and-forth movement of the soft brain within the bony skull in a brain injury.

divided attention. The mechanism by which the brain maintains focus on more than one task at a time.

electroencephalogram (EEG). A recording of the electrical activity in the brain.

epidural hematoma. A collection of blood right below the skull, between the skull and the dura mater, the outermost covering of the brain.

executive function. The ability to set a goal, initiate action toward the goal, monitor progress toward the goal, and modify the course if necessary to achieve the goal.

family therapy. A form of psychotherapy that focuses on the entire family and in which each family member participates.

generalized anxiety disorder (GAD). A medical diagnosis of persistent free-floating anxiety for prolonged periods that interferes with a person's everyday activities.

generalized seizure. A seizure in which the entire brain is affected, often leading to loss of consciousness and jerking movements throughout the body. There are many types of generalized seizures, such as tonic-clonic (also known as grand-mal), atonic, myoclonic, and absence seizures.

grand-mal seizure. *See* generalized seizure.

gray matter. A type of brain tissue that contains neurons.

group therapy. A form of psychotherapy in which a small number of people with similar issues meet regularly with a therapist to discuss their problems and discuss ways they have dealt with their problems.

hallucinations. Sensory experiences of hearing, seeing, feeling, or smelling things when there are no external stimuli.

hematoma. A blood clot or a collection of blood outside a blood vessel.

hemorrhage. Active bleeding.

illogical thinking. A pattern of thinking in psychosis in which thoughts are jumbled or disorganized; a form of psychosis.

impact injury. Injury that occurs when the head makes sudden, forceful contact with some object.

impulsivity. Acting on a whim without consideration of the consequences.

injury from inertial forces. Injury that results when the brain moves within the skull, but not as a result of impact to the head.

insomnia. The inability to fall asleep or stay asleep.

interpersonal therapy (IPT). A form of psychotherapy whose goal is to help the patient improve interpersonal skills and either resolve or cope with interpersonal problems.

intracerebral hemorrhage. Bleeding within the soft tissue of the brain.

intracranial hemorrhage. Bleeding within the head, either between the skull and the brain or within the soft tissue of the brain.

magnetic resonance imaging (MRI). An imaging technique that uses a magnetic field to obtain pictures of the body's soft tissues.

mania. A prolonged state of heightened mental and physical activity leading to impairment of day-to-day functioning.

memory. A collection of processes that lead to learning and recalling information.

narcolepsy. A condition in which the person experiences episodes of sudden and uncontrollable sleep.

neuromuscular junction. A gap between a neuron and a muscle cell.

neuron. A brain cell; the brain's fundamental unit of operation.

neurotransmitters. Chemicals within the brain that help in communication between brain cells.

nonepileptic seizure. A type of spell that appears to be a seizure but without evidence of seizure on an EEG.

panic attack. A sudden wave of anxiety that occurs without warning, often with prominent physical symptoms such as heart racing or shortness of breath. A panic attack can be so severe that the person experiencing it may think he or she is about to die.

partial seizure. A seizure that affects only one part of the brain, and there is not complete loss of consciousness.

penetrating injury. An injury sustained when an object penetrates the soft tissue of the brain.

posttraumatic stress disorder (PTSD). An anxiety disorder that develops after exposure to a stressful and traumatic event. The person with PTSD can re-experience the trauma in flashbacks or nightmares.

psychosis. Gross distortion of reality, with disorganized emotional responses and impairment of day-to-day functioning.

reticular activating system (RAS). A network within the brain that is responsible for consciousness and alertness.

seizure. An abnormal amount of electrical discharge in either part of the brain or the entire brain that can produce body movements, alteration of awareness, or sensory changes.

selective attention. The mechanism by which the brain chooses which stimuli in the environment to engage with. It involves the ability to inhibit the processing of distractions.

serotonin-norepinephrine reuptake inhibitors (SNRIs). Medications that increase the brain chemicals norepinephrine and serotonin. SNRIs are often used to treat depression.

selective serotonin reuptake inhibitors (SSRIs). Medications that increase the brain chemical serotonin. SSRIs are often used to treat depression.

sleep apnea. A condition of abnormal breathing while sleeping, leading to a cessation of breathing while sleeping. Sleep apnea is associated with daytime sleepiness.

soma. The main body of a neuron (brain cell).

subarachnoid hemorrhage. A collection of blood closer to the brain than a subdural hematoma, but still outside the brain. Subarachnoid hemorrhages develop below the arachnoid mater but beneath the dura mater.

subdural hematoma. A collection of blood between the brain and the skull, but below the dura mater. Subdural hematomas are closer to the brain than epidural hematomas, but still outside the brain.

sustained attention, or vigilance. The mechanism by which the brain maintains focus on something for a longer period of time than required for selective attention.

synapse. The space between any two neurons where electrochemical signals are transferred from one neuron to the other.

tonic-clonic seizure. *See* generalized seizure.

traumatic brain injury (TBI). A brain injury caused by physical trauma.

white matter. A type of brain tissue that contains nerve fibers, mostly axons, which carry signals to different parts of the brain.

RESOURCES

We provide a number of resources for people with brain injuries and their families and for professionals. The stated missions and goals of the organizations mentioned here were taken directly from their websites to capture accurately what they have to offer.

TBI Advocacy Organizations

Brain Injury Association of America (BIAA)
http://www.biausa.org/
> The mission of BIAA is to promote "brain injury prevention, research, treatment and education and to improve the quality of life for all people affected by brain injury." The organization has a network of state affiliates that provide support, education, resources, and advocacy for persons with brain injury and their friends and family.

National Association of State Head Injury Administrators (NASHIA)
http://www.nashia.org/
> NASHIA's mission is to assist state government in promoting partnerships and building systems to meet the needs of individuals with brain injury and their families. NASHIA collaborates with TBI stakeholders and organizations such as BIAA and the National Disability Rights Network (NDRN) to revise and regulate brain injury policies and promote funding.

TBI-related Clinical Activities, Education, and Research

Centers for Disease Control and Prevention
http://www.cdc.gov/concussion/index.html
> Centers for Disease Control and Prevention offer information and educational materials for physicians and coaches on concussion and concussion prevention.

The Brain Injury Guide and Resources
http://www.braininjuryeducation.org/
> This online resource is a collaboration of the Missouri Department of Health and Senior Services and the MU Department of Health Psychology. It is a valuable site for those seeking to cope with and understand TBI.

National Resource Center for Traumatic Brain Injury (NRCTBI)
http://www.tbinrc.com/
The mission of NRCTBI is to provide relevant, practical information for persons with brain injury, their family members, and professionals. It is located at the Virginia Commonwealth University's Medical College of Virginia campus, and many of the staff of NRCTBI are associated with the Virginia Commonwealth TBI Model System.

The Traumatic Brain Injury Model Systems (TBIMS) program
http://www.msktc.org/tbi/model-system-centers
TBIMS program is sponsored by the National Institute on Disability and Rehabilitation Research. The program supports research projects focused on "delivery, demonstration, and evaluation of medical, rehabilitation, vocational, and other services designed to meet the needs of individuals with traumatic brain injury." Grants are awarded to institutions that are leaders in TBI care and research.

Brain Injury Resource Center
http://www.headinjury.com/
Brain Injury Resource Center is a nonprofit clearinghouse founded and operated by brain injury activists. The goal of their website is to share their experiences with the intention of helping decrease the grief and suffering that individuals with brain injury go through and to promote proactive involvement, knowledge, self-awareness, and self-advocacy following brain injury.

Ohio Valley Center for Brain Injury Prevention and Rehabilitation
http://www.ohiovalley.org/
The mission of Ohio Valley Center for Brain Injury Prevention and Rehabilitation is to conduct research, provide education, and develop programs to improve the quality of life of persons who experience traumatic brain injury. The organization serves individuals with TBI, families, and professionals throughout the United States.

UAB-TBIMS Home Stimulation Program
https://www.uab.edu/medicine/tbi/uab-tbi-information-network/uab
-tbims-home-based-cognitive-stimulation-activities
UAB-TBIMS Home Stimulation Program has been developed by the University of Alabama Traumatic Brain Injury Model System. It provides activities for individuals with brain injury and their family members and caregivers. These activities are tailored to help improve cognitive skills and assist individuals in recovering their thinking skill.

LEARNet

> http://www.projectlearnet.org/
> LEARNet is an online resource for teachers, clinicians, parents, and students developed by the Brain Injury Association of New York State. The website provides problem-solving techniques to help students with brain injury at home and school.

Michigan Traumatic Brain Injury Online Training

> http://www.mitbitraining.org/
> Michigan Traumatic Brain Injury Online Training is an online training site that provides training courses with the goal of educating people and promoting awareness of the causes, symptoms, and treatment of TBI. This training can be helpful to persons with TBI, their family members, caregivers, professionals, policy makers, and the general public.

AbleData

> http://www.abledata.com/abledata.cfm?CFID=27570632&CFTOKEN =20d4f90799a4b620-3254342B-E3AB-7D5A-D554B56791848DAD
> The AbleData website provides information on different types of assistive technology available to people with all types of disability. The website does not sell products, but it helps people locate companies that do.

Lash and Associates Publishing/Training, Inc.

> http://www.lapublishing.com/
> Lash and Associates Publishing/Training, Inc. offers information on TBI and posttraumatic stress disorder (PTSD) in the form of books, tip cards, manuals, and tool kits that can be used in hospitals, rehabilitation programs, community agencies, schools, private practice, and at home. People who can benefit from visiting this site include people with brain injury, their families, and professionals.

Employment-focused Resources

Job Accommodation Network

> https://askjan.org/links/about.htm
> https://askjan.org/media/BrainInjury.html#info
> Job Accommodation Network (JAN) is a comprehensive job accommodation resource. It provides people with disabilities guidance on workplace accommodations. JAN is one of several services provided by the US Department of Labor's Office of Disability Employment Policy (ODEP). It has been built through the collaborative efforts of ODEP, West Virginia University, and private industry throughout North America.

Military-based Resources
BrainLineMilitary

    http://www.brainlinemilitary.org/

    BrainLineMilitary is an online TBI resource guide for service members, veterans, national guards, and their families. The site provides information on military TBI, resources, personal stories, research updates, and topics by health care professionals who treat military members with traumatic brain injuries.

Defense and Veterans Brain Injury Center (DVBIC)

    http://dvbic.dcoe.mil/

    DVBIC is a part of the US military health system. Its mission is to serve active duty military, their families, and veterans with TBI. It fulfills its mission through ongoing collaboration with the Department of Defense, military services, Department of Veterans Affairs, civilian health partners, and individuals with TBI.

America's Heroes at Work

    http://www.americasheroesatwork.gov/

    This website was created to assist veterans with TBI and posttraumatic stress disorder (PTSD), but it is useful for civilians too. It is geared toward potential employers and can be used when educating an employer or potential employers about brain injury. A project of the US Department of Labor, it addresses work-related challenges of returning service members and veterans who have sustained a TBI or have PTSD, or both.

Veterans Health Information Clearing House

    https://www.health.ny.gov/health_care/veterans/

    Veterans Health Information Clearing House provides a list of resources for veterans, their families, and health care providers on illnesses that may be service connected, as well as a list of the various available federal and state health care services.

SUGGESTED READING

General Interest Books about the Brain

Nancy L. Mace and Peter V. Rabins, *The 36-Hour Day: A Family Guide to Caring for Persons with Alzheimer Disease, Related Dementing Illnesses, and Memory Loss in Later Life.*

Anjan Chatterjee, *The Aesthetic Brain: How We Evolved to Desire Beauty and Enjoy Art.*

V. S. Ramachandran and Sandra Blakeslee, *Phantoms in the Brain: Probing the Mysteries of the Human Mind.*

Stephen Pinker, *How the Mind Works.*

Books for Professionals

David B. Arciniegas, Nathan D. Zasler, Rodney D. Vanderploeg, and Michael S. Jaffee, eds., *Management of Adults with Traumatic Brain Injury.*

Jonathan M. Silver, Thomas W. McAllister, and Stuart C. Yudofsky, *Textbook of Traumatic Brain Injury.*

Articles

T. W. McAllister, Neurobiological consequences of traumatic brain injury, *Dialogues in Clinical Neuroscience* 13.3 (2011): 287–300.

J. M. Silver, Neuropsychiatry of persistent symptoms after concussion, *Psychiatric Clinics of North America* 37.1 (2014): 91–102.

R. E. Jorge and D. B Arciniegas, Mood disorders after TBI, *Psychiatric Clinics of North America* 37.1 (2014): 13–29.

I

INDEX

Abilify (aripiprazole), 85
AbleData website, 187
acetaminophen (Tylenol), 29, 152
acetylcholine: in aggression, 94; in
  delirium, 84; drug effects on, 77,
  91, 123, 130, 131, 137; in sleep
  disturbances, 109
acetylcholinesterase inhibitors, 77,
  123, 130, 137, 145
Adderall (dextroamphetamine),
  76–77, 123, 130, 137
adrenaline, 46
adrenocorticotropic hormone
  (ACTH), 58
advanced sleep phase syndrome, 111
advocacy organizations, 185
aggression, 79, 89–98, 179; brain
  circuitry of, 92–93; delirium and,
  60; depression and, 43; mania and,
  67, 68; risk factors and triggers for,
  90, 97; symptoms and causes of,
  90–94; timing of, 91; treatment of,
  90, 91, 94–95
agitation, 120, 122; aggression and,
  89, 90; anxiety and, 61; in delirium,
  60; Depakote (valproic acid) for, 153;
  drug-induced, 61, 92, 160; language
  problems and, 144; mania and, 70;
  pain and, 92; psychosis and, 82, 85,
  86, 87, 88
alcohol use, 176; aggression and, 90,
  97; apathy and, 76; cerebellar effect
  of, 18; depression and, 43, 46, 54–55;
  executive function and, 138;

impulsivity and, 101–2; language
  problems and, 145; mania and, 69,
  70, 71; recovery and, 32; sleep
  problems and, 109, 116; subdural
  hematoma and, 25; withdrawal
  from, 62, 91, 92, 162
alprazolam (Xanax), 32, 91, 114
Alzheimer's disease, 19, 35, 46, 74,
  127, 130, 131
amantadine, 77, 103–4, 123, 131, 137
Ambien (zolpidem), 114
America's Heroes at Work, 188
amphetamines, 85, 92
amygdala, 17, 19, 44, 45, 58, 59, 68,
  73, 93, 100, 158
anemia, 74, 84, 112
anger, 55, 61, 66, 90, 92, 97, 100, 142,
  144, 157
anomia, 140, 141–42, 143, 144, 179
anoxic injury, 24, 26
anterior cingulate, 17, 19–20, 44, 73,
  121, 135
antidepressants, 47–49, 51, 75, 77,
  96, 131
antihistamines, 109
antipsychotics, 49, 67, 69, 85–86,
  91, 96
antiseizure medications, 81, 96, 104,
  153, 155, 159, 160–61, 162
Anton's syndrome, 166
anxiety, 20, 29, 30, 57–65, 179; brain
  circuitry of, 57–59; depression
  and, 43, 53, 57; drug-induced, 62;
  hallucinations and, 82; impact on

anxiety (cont.)
    recovery, 31–32, 34; seizures and, 157–58; symptoms of, 59–62; tips for coping with, 63–65; treatment of, 62–63, 64
apathy, 72–78, 179; brain circuitry of, 73; depression and, 73, 74–75, 77; diagnosis of, 75; drug-induced, 76, 78; medical causes of, 74; symptoms of, 73–75; tips for coping with, 77–78; treatment of, 75–77
Apathy Evaluation Scale, 75
aphasia, 140–44, 179; fluent (jargon), 141–42, 143, 144; global (total), 142; nonfluent, 141, 142, 143, 144. See also language problems
appetite changes, 42, 45, 74
aprosody, 142, 144, 179
Aricept (donepezil), 77, 123, 130, 131, 137, 145
aripiprazole (Abilify), 85
arousal, 119–20, 121, 123, 179
assault, 89, 155. See also aggression
Ativan (lorazepam), 32, 62, 91, 95, 114
attention, 179; divided, 119, 120–21, 180; memory and, 121, 126, 127; selective, 119, 120, 121, 182; sustained, 119, 120, 183
attention deficit hyperactivity disorder (ADHD), 124, 130–31
attention problems, 2, 30, 31, 119–24; brain circuitry of, 121; tips for coping with, 123–24; treatment of, 122–23
attention training, 122
auditory processing, 16, 19
autonomic nervous system, 10
axons, 10–12, 26, 179; diffuse axonal injury, 26–28, 109, 180; retinal, 165
axon tracts, 15, 16, 73, 84

balance problems, 18, 163
basal ganglia, 15, 17, 18, 68, 73, 76, 85, 121
"bath salts," 85
behavioral interventions, 3, 4, 8, 30; for aggression, 94–95; for apathy, 76; for attention problems, 122; for depression, 51; for executive dysfunction, 136–37; for impulsivity, 102–3; for mania, 69; for memory problems, 129–30. See also cognitive behavioral therapy; dialectical behavioral therapy
behavioral problems, 2, 4, 23, 33, 47, 79–116; ABCs of assessment for, 94–95; aggression, 89–98; impulsivity, 99–105; psychosis, 81–88; sleep disturbances, 106–16
Benadryl (diphenhydramine), 91
benzodiazepines, 62, 95, 114; withdrawal from, 91–92, 95
beta blockers, 96
biofeedback, 51
biological clock, 109
bipolar disorder: depression in, 41, 43, 49; mania in, 66–71
blast injury, 21, 22, 26, 179
bleeding in the brain, 2, 24–25, 26, 28, 35, 39, 59, 66, 92, 99, 151, 158
blindness, 3, 20, 166
Botox (botulinum toxin) injections, 152–53
brain damage, types of, 22–28; bleeding in brain, 24–25; bruises, cuts, and skull fractures, 22–24; neuronal damage, 26–28; oxygen deprivation, 26; pressure on brain, 25–26
brain herniation, 26
Brain Injury Association of America (BIAA), 185
The Brain Injury Guide and Resources, 185
Brain Injury Resource Center, 186
BrainLineMilitary website, 188
brain plasticity, 28, 30, 124, 131, 144
brainstem, 10, 16–17
brain structure and function, 7–20; cellular, 10–12; circuitry, 12–14; illustrations of, 16, 17; white matter and gray matter, 15. See also specific structures

brain swelling, 22, 35, 39, 106
brain-training programs, 124
breathing, 10, 16, 26
breathing exercises, 64, 103
bright-light therapy, 113
Broca's area, 143
bromocriptine, 76, 131
bruising of brain, 22–23, 180
buddy system, 55, 132, 162
bupropion (Wellbutrin), 48, 77
BuSpar (buspirone), 96

caffeine, 55, 152, 154
calling 911 for help, 56, 70, 87, 97, 151,
    155, 157, 161, 175
car accidents, 1, 22, 25, 26, 29, 57, 89,
    92, 125, 140, 164, 171
carbamazepine (Tegretol), 49, 69, 96,
    104, 161
carbidopa-levodopa (Sinemet), 77
catastrophic thinking, 32, 34
caudate, 18
Celexa (citalopram), 47, 62, 96
Centers for Disease Control and
    Prevention, 185
central nervous system, 9–10
cerebellum, 10, 16, 17, 18
cerebral cortex, 10, 18
chronic traumatic encephalopathy
    (CTE), 33, 179
circadian rhythm disorder, 106–7,
    111–12, 113–14, 179
citalopram (Celexa), 47, 62, 96
clonazepam (Klonopin), 62, 91,
    114
cocaine, 32, 62, 85, 92
cognitive behavioral therapy (CBT),
    51, 62–63, 94, 152, 180
cognitive exercise, 54, 122, 124
cognitive functioning, 17, 18–19
cognitive problems, 2, 4, 19, 29,
    117; attention, 119–24; executive
    function, 133–39; language disor-
    ders, 140–46; memory, 125–32;
    after mild TBI, 30, 31; after severe
    TBI, 35
cognitive "prosthetics," 130, 132

cognitive rehabilitation, 35, 122, 130,
    136–37
cognitive tests, 29, 30
coma, 26, 39, 120, 121, 133, 155
combat injuries, 1, 22, 26, 61, 163, 179
compliance with therapy, 174, 175
compulsive behaviors, 81
computerized tomography (CT) scan,
    28, 29, 149, 180
concentration problems, 31, 40, 42,
    47, 106, 107, 119. See also attention
    problems
concussion. See mild TBI
confusion, 17, 28, 149; aggression
    and, 91, 120; in delirium, 60–61,
    84, 91, 120; drug-induced, 77; in
    psychosis, 86; seizures and, 156,
    157, 158
consciousness, 9, 12, 16, 29, 182;
    delirium and, 60, 84; loss of, 1, 16,
    28, 39, 61, 89, 149, 171; seizures and,
    156, 158, 161, 181, 182
contusion of brain, 22–23, 125, 171, 180
conversion disorder, 159
coordination circuits, 12
corticospinal tract, 12
cortisol, 46, 49
cortisol-releasing factor (CRF), 58
coup-contrecoup injury, 23, 180
crying, 44, 110
Cymbalta (duloxetine), 150

dangerous behavior, 68, 69, 102
deep brain stimulation, 20, 50, 177
Defense and Veterans Brain Injury
    Center (DVBIC), 188
delayed sleep phase syndrome, 106–7,
    111–12
delirium, 60–61; aggression and, 91,
    92, 95; drug-induced, 77, 84, 91;
    inattention and, 120; psychosis
    and, 84, 85
delusions, 82, 84, 85, 86, 180; depres-
    sion and, 43; epilepsy and, 159;
    mania and, 67; paranoid, 81, 82;
    persecutory, 85; treatment of,
    85–86

dendrites, 10–12, 180
Depakote (valproic acid), 49, 67, 69, 96, 104, 153, 161
depersonalization, 158
depression, 20, 30, 37, 39–56, 172, 173; acceptance as normal after TBI, 42, 53; alcohol or drug use and, 43; anxiety and, 43, 53, 57; apathy and, 73, 74–75, 77; bipolar, 41, 43, 49; brain circuitry of, 44–46; clinical (major), 40–41, 179–80; impact on recovery, 32, 43, 46; life stressors and, 48–49; migraine and, 153; after mild TBI, 31–32; mimics of, 43–44; risk factors for, 41; spectrum of, 41; suicide and, 41, 42–43, 47, 53, 56, 75; symptoms of, 41–43; tips for coping with, 53–56; treatment of, 46–53, 172, 177
desensitization, 51
desvenlafaxine (Pristiq), 48, 77
dextroamphetamine (Adderall), 76–77, 123, 130, 137
dextromethorphan/quinidine (Nuedexta), 49
dialectical behavioral therapy (DBT), 52, 180
diazepam (Valium), 32, 62, 114
diet, 54, 55, 70, 103, 152, 154, 172
diffuse axonal injury (DAI), 26–28, 109, 180
diffusion tensor imaging (DTI), 28
Dilantin (phenytoin), 160
diphenhydramine (Benadryl), 91
disorientation, 17, 28, 29, 91, 120, 125, 149
Ditropan (oxybutynin), 91
dizziness, 28, 30, 31, 61, 151, 153–54
DNA, 14
donepezil (Aricept), 77, 123, 130, 131, 137, 145
dopamine, 12; in aggression, 94–95; in depression, 47–49; drugs affecting levels of, 86, 94, 104; in mania, 68; in motivation, 75–76
driving after TBI, 123, 162, 173, 176
drugs. See medications

drug use. See illicit drug use
duloxetine (Cymbalta), 150
dysgraphia, 141

Ecstasy, 85
Effexor (venlafaxine), 48, 62, 77
Eldepryl (selegiline), 77, 131
electroconvulsive therapy (ECT), 50
electroencephalogram (EEG), 85, 159, 160, 180
eletriptan (Relpax), 152
embarrassment, 61, 91, 105, 176
emotional brain. See limbic system
emotional problems, 2–5, 37; anxiety, 57–65; apathy, 72–78; depression, 39–56; mania, 66–71
emotional trauma, 2
emotions, 9, 13; expression in speech, 142; impact on recovery from mild TBI, 31–32, 34; pseudobulbar affect, 44, 49; regulation of, 16, 17, 19, 20
employment, 2, 187; depression and, 40; return to work, 119, 122, 171–72; shift work, 70–71, 108, 112; vocational rehabilitation, 122
environmental factors: genetics and, 14; sleep and, 109, 110
environmental interventions: for aggression, 94–95, 96; for apathy, 76; for attention problems, 122; for cognitive problems, 136; for executive dysfunction, 136; for impulsivity, 102; for memory problems, 129–30; for sleep problems, 114; for visual problems, 169
epilepsy, 156, 158–59, 161
escitalopram (Lexapro), 47, 62, 96, 104
eszopiclone (Lunesta), 114
euphoria, 67, 70
excessive daytime sleepiness, 106, 110–11
executive function, 16, 19, 120, 134, 180
executive function deficits, 133–39; brain circuitry of, 134, 135; symptoms of, 134–36; tips for coping with, 138–39; treatment of, 136–38

Exelon (rivastigmine), 77, 130
exercise, 33; for apathy, 76; for depression, 32, 46, 53–54, 55, 172; for headaches, 152, 154; to improve sleep, 115; for mania, 70
exposure therapy, 51

falls, 1, 22, 25, 39, 72, 89, 92, 99, 106, 133, 161
family/caregivers, 2, 33, 35–36, 174–75; and patient's aggression, 96–98; and patient's anxiety, 64–65; and patient's apathy, 74, 77; and patient's depression, 55–56; and patient's executive dysfunction, 138–30; and patient's impulsivity, 104–5; and patient's language problems, 145–46; and patient's mania, 70–71; and patient's memory problems, 131, 132; and patient's psychosis, 86–88; and patient's seizures, 161–62; and patient's sleep problems, 114–15
family therapy, 52, 181
fatigue, 54, 107, 112, 130, 138, 171
Fetzima (levomilnacipran), 48
fight-or-flight response, 58, 59, 93
flashbacks, 34, 61
fluoxetine (Prozac), 47
frontal lobes, 16, 18–19; activation by neuromodulation therapy, 50; aggression and, 92, 93; apathy and, 73; bleeding in, 25, 39; contusion of, 23–24, 125; depression and, 45–46, 48; executive function and, 134, 135; impulsivity and, 100, 101, 103, 104; language and, 142, 143; mania and, 68; memory and, 128; psychosis and, 85; seizures in, 157, 158; vision and, 166
frustration, 34, 61, 84, 149, 172, 175; due to language problems, 140, 141, 142, 144, 146; due to memory loss, 125, 131, 132; due to sleep problems, 107, 111; of family, 74, 81, 94

gabapentin (Neurontin), 161
galantamine (Razadyne), 77, 130
gamma-aminobutyric acid (GABA), 12, 94
generalized anxiety disorder (GAD), 59–60, 181
genetics, 14
glial cells, 10
globus pallidus, 18
glossary, 7, 179–83
glutamate, 12; amantadine effects on, 104, 123, 131, 137
gray matter of brain, 15, 181
group therapy, 52–53, 181
growth hormone, 18
guilty feelings, 42, 61, 74
gunshot injury, 22, 24

Haldol (haloperidol), 85
hallucinations, 82–83, 84, 181; during alcohol or benzodiazepine withdrawal, 92; auditory, 19, 82–83; delirium and, 60; depression and, 43; mania and, 67; treatment of, 85–86
headaches, 28, 29, 30, 61, 149–54, 171; symptoms and types of, 151–52; TBI and, 150; tips for coping with, 154; treatment of, 152–54; triggers for, 154
hematoma, 24, 181; epidural, 24, 25, 180; subdural, 24–25, 171, 183
hemorrhage, 24, 181; intracerebral, 25, 181; intracranial, 24, 181; subarachnoid, 24, 25, 183
heroin, 32, 62
higher-order brain circuits, 12–13
hippocampus, 19, 44, 45, 49, 85, 128
hope for future, 176–78
hopelessness, 42, 72, 74, 75
hostility, 55, 89
hydrocodone/acetaminophen (Vicodin), 32, 92
hypersomnia, posttraumatic, 111
hypomania, 68
hypothalamus, 15, 17, 45, 58, 59, 93, 108

ibuprofen (Motrin), 151, 152
illicit drug use, 176; aggression and, 90, 92, 97; anxiety and, 62; apathy and, 76, 78; depression and, 43, 46, 54–55; executive function and, 138; impact on recovery, 32; impulsivity and, 101–2; language problems and, 145; mania and, 69, 70; psychosis and, 85; sleep problems and, 116
illogical thinking, 82, 83, 181
Imitrex (sumatriptan), 149, 152
impact injury, 21–22, 181
impulsivity, 3, 58, 79, 99–105, 181; aggression and, 90; brain circuitry of, 100; mania and, 67, 68; symptoms and causes of, 100–102; tips for coping with, 104–5; treatment of, 102–4
Inderal (propranolol), 96, 153
inertial forces injury, 21, 22, 26, 181
inflammation, 26, 46, 48, 49
insomnia, 106, 107, 110, 171, 181.
See also sleep disturbances
interpersonal therapy (IPT), 52, 181
irritability, 30, 34, 43, 61, 67, 68

Job Accommodation Network, 187

Keppra (levetiracetam), 160
Klonopin (clonazepam), 62, 91, 114

laceration of brain, 24
Lamictal (lamotrigine), 49, 160–61
language problems, 28, 140–46; brain circuitry of, 142–43; symptoms of, 141–43; tips for coping with, 145–46; treatment of, 143–45. See also anomia; aphasia
Lash and Associates Publishing/ Training, Inc., 187
Latuda (lurasidone), 49, 85
"laziness," 72, 74, 77, 138
LEARNet, 187
left hemisphere of brain, 46, 142
levetiracetam (Keppra), 160
levodopa, 77, 131
levomilnacipran (Fetzima), 48

Lexapro (escitalopram), 47, 62, 96, 104
limbic system, 19; in aggression, 93; in depression, 44–45, 48–49; in impulsivity, 100
lithium, 49, 69
litigation/compensation issues, 33, 34
locked-in syndrome, 16–17
lorazepam (Ativan), 32, 62, 91, 95, 114
LSD, 85
Lunesta (eszopiclone), 114
lurasidone (Latuda), 49, 85

magnetic resonance imaging (MRI), 28, 29, 85, 182
magnetic seizure therapy, 50
mamillary body, 19
mania, 37, 43, 66–71, 182; double-hit theory of, 68; symptoms of, 67–68; tips for coping with, 70–71; treatment of, 69
marijuana, 32, 74, 76, 78, 85, 176
medical advocate/companion, 174
medical records, 173
medications, 3, 4; for aggression, 90, 95–96; for anxiety, 62, 64; for apathy, 76–77; for attention problems, 123; cautions for use of, 5; compliance with, 174, 175; for depression, 47–49, 172; for executive function deficits, 137; for headaches, 149, 152–53; for language disorders, 145; for mania, 669; for memory problems, 130–31; for seizures, 81, 96, 104, 153, 155, 159, 160–61, 162; for sleep disturbances, 114. See also specific medications and classes
meditation, 34, 35, 51, 63, 64, 103, 150, 152, 154. See also mindfulness meditation
medulla, 16
melatonin, 113
memory(ies), 126–27, 182; attention and, 121, 126, 127; episodic, 126–27; explicit, 126; formation of, 1, 19, 85; implicit, 126, 127; metamemory, 127; regulation of, 3, 12, 14, 16, 17,

19; retrieval of, 127; semantic, 126, 127; short- and long-term, 127, 134; storage of, 19, 127, 128; working, 127, 134

memory problems, 2, 13, 30, 31, 125–32; assessment of, 128; brain circuitry of, 128; tips for coping with, 132; treatment of, 129–31

methamphetamine, 85

methylphenidate (Ritalin), 76, 96, 123, 130, 131, 137, 145

Michigan Traumatic Brain Injury Online Training, 187

midbrain, 16

migraine, 151, 152–53

mild TBI, 1–2, 21, 29–30, 149; due to diffuse axonal injury, 28; persistent symptoms after, 30, 31; recovery from, 30–34

military-based resources, 188

mindfulness meditation, 51, 52, 150, 154

moderate to severe TBI, 1–2; factors affecting recovery from, 30, 34–35. See also severe TBI

monoamine oxidase type A (MAO-A), 94

mood stabilizers, 49, 67, 69

mood symptoms, 2, 30, 37; anxiety, 57–65; apathy, 72–78; depression, 39–56; impact on recovery, 31–32, 34; mania, 66–71

motivation, 12, 17, 19, 72; depression and, 47; dopamine and, 75–76; executive function and, 134, 135, 136; lack of, 72, 73, 77–78, 175 (see also apathy); language problems and, 143; psychosis and, 84; sleep problems and, 110

motor circuits, 12

motor cortex, 16, 19

Motrin (ibuprofen), 151, 152

music, 54, 76

myelin, 15

napping, 54, 115

narcolepsy, 110–11, 112, 115, 182

National Association of State Head Injury Administrators (NASHIA), 185

National Resource Center for Traumatic Brain Injury (NRCTBI), 186

nervous system, 9–10

neurological examination, 29

neuromodulation therapy, 20, 49–50, 177–78

neuromuscular junction, 10, 182

neurons, 10–12, 15, 182; damage to, 26–28

Neurontin (gabapentin), 161

neuropsychological tests. See cognitive tests

neurotransmitters, 12, 182; in aggression, 93–94; in apathy, 75–76; in depression, 47–49; in mania, 68. See also specific neurotransmitters

new baseline. See personality, changes in

"new normal," 35

nightmares, 34, 92, 95

nonepileptic seizures (NES), 159–60, 182

nonrapid eye movement (NREM) sleep, 108–9, 112

norepinephrine (noradrenaline), 12; in aggression, 93–94; in anxiety, 58; in depression, 47–49; drugs affecting levels of, 48, 94, 123, 130, 137, 183; in mania, 68; in sleep disturbances, 109

nucleus accumbens, 18

Nuedexta (dextromethorphan/ quinidine), 49

occipital lobes, 16, 18; contusion of, 23; seizures in, 157; vision and, 20, 165–66

occipital neuralgia, 151

occupational therapy (OT), 35, 39, 55, 76, 78, 102, 122, 133, 137, 172, 174

Ohio Valley Center for Brain Injury Prevention and Rehabilitation, 186

olanzapine (Zyprexa), 69, 85

omega-3 fatty acids, 54, 103
optic nerve damage, 164–68
orbitofrontal cortex, 17, 19, 92, 93, 100, 135
oxybutynin (Ditropan), 91
oxycodone/acetaminophen (Percocet), 32, 92
OxyContin (oxycodone), 92

pain. See headaches
pain medications: aggression and, 91, 92; apathy and, 76; headaches due to overuse of, 151, 152, 154; misuse or abuse of, 32; withdrawal from, 92
panic attacks, 60, 157–58, 182
paranoia, 81, 82
paraphasias, 141
parasympathetic nervous system, 10
parietal lobes, 16, 18; anomia and, 143; seizures in, 157; selective attention and, 121; vision and, 166, 167
Parkinson's disease, 18, 35, 73, 74, 103, 131
pathological laughing and crying, 44
PCP, 92
penetrating injury, 21, 22, 26, 158, 182
Percocet (oxycodone/acetaminophen), 32, 92
periodic limb movement disorder, 112
peripheral nervous system, 9–10
personality: changes in, 19, 23, 58–59, 68, 73–74, 99, 101; impact on recovery, 32
pharmacogenetic testing, 176–77
phenytoin (Dilantin), 160
physical therapy (PT), 35, 39, 72, 136–37, 171, 174
pituitary gland, 17–18, 58
polysomnography (PSG), 112
pons, 16, 108
positive reinforcement, 103, 104, 137, 138–39, 175
post concussion syndrome. See mild TBI

posttraumatic stress disorder (PTSD), 33, 34, 61, 92, 150, 182
prefrontal cortex, 16, 19; dorsolateral, 17, 19, 73, 121, 128, 135; medial, 17, 19, 135; ventral, 19, 135
premotor cortex, 16, 19
pressure in the brain, 25–26, 150
Pristiq (desvenlafaxine), 48, 77
problem-solving training, 76
propranolol (Inderal), 96, 153
Prozac (fluoxetine), 47
pseudobulbar affect (PBA), 44, 49
psychiatric symptoms, 2–5
psychosis, 79, 81–88, 182; brain circuitry of, 84–85; risk factors for, 83–85; symptoms of, 82–83; timing of, 84, 86; tips for coping with, 87–88; treatment of, 85–86
psychotherapy, 34, 35, 62–63, 64, 69, 76, 113, 152, 174; for aggression, 94; for anxiety, 62–63; for depression, 46, 50–53; for headaches, 152; for mania, 69. See also specific types of psychotherapy
putamen, 18

quality of life, 2, 32, 35, 37, 159, 167
quetiapine (Seroquel), 49, 67, 69, 85

ramelteon (Rozerem), 114
rapid eye movement (REM) sleep, 108–9, 112
Razadyne (galantamine), 77, 130
recovery, 29–36, 171–78; anxiety and, 31–32, 34; depression and, 32, 43, 46; drug or alcohol use and, 32; legal issues and, 34; from mild TBI, 30–34; from moderate to severe TBI, 34–35; personality and, 32; previous TBIs and, 33; severity of injury and, 30, 35; social support and, 33–34
rehabilitation, 30, 35, 39; cognitive, 35, 122, 130, 136–37; visual, 167–68; vocational, 122
relaxation training, 51, 114, 154
Relpax (eletriptan), 152

REM sleep behavior disorder, 108
repeat TBIs, 2, 33, 90
resources, 185–88
rest, 33, 54, 76, 124, 129–30, 149
restless legs syndrome (RLS), 112
reticular activating system (RAS), 16, 121, 182
right hemisphere of brain, 121, 142
Risperdal (risperidone), 69, 85
Ritalin (methylphenidate), 76, 96, 123, 130, 131, 137, 145
ritualistic behaviors, 81
rivastigmine (Exelon), 77, 130
Rozerem (ramelteon), 114

sadness, 39–44, 51, 72, 74, 75, 157, 172
safety precautions, 56, 70, 87, 90, 97, 161–62, 175
schizophrenia, 19, 73, 83–84, 85, 141. *See also* psychosis
scotomas, 166
scripts, behavioral, 137, 139
seizures, 2, 28, 155–62, 182; aggression and, 89, 92; complex partial, 157, 158, 180; duration of, 156; epilepsy, 156, 158–59, 161; generalized, 156–57, 161, 181; grand-mal, 156, 181; intracerebral hemorrhage and, 25; nonepileptic, 159–60, 182; partial, 156, 157–58, 161, 182; penetrating injury and, 22, 26; psychosis and, 81, 83, 85; risk factors for, 158; after severe TBI, 81, 83, 85, 92, 155, 158, 160, 161; skull fracture and, 24; timing of, 155–56, 158, 160; tips for coping with, 161–62; tonic-clonic, 156–57, 183; treatment of, 160–61; triggers for, 162
selective serotonin reuptake inhibitors (SSRIs), 47–48, 49, 62, 76, 177, 183
selegiline (Eldepryl), 77, 131
self-care, 39
self-regulation, 100, 102, 103, 104, 137
self-treatment, 3
sense of self, 9, 35, 117
sensitivity to light or sound, 30, 92, 152, 167

sensory circuits, 12
Seroquel (quetiapine), 49, 67, 69, 85
serotonin, 12; in aggression, 93–94; in bipolar disorder, 68; in depression, 47–49; drugs affecting levels of, 47, 48, 62, 74, 92, 104, 153, 177, 183; in sleep disturbances, 109
serotonin norepinephrine reuptake inhibitors (SNRIs), 48, 62, 104, 183
sertraline (Zoloft), 4, 47, 62, 96, 104
severe TBI, 1–2, 72, 81; aggression after, 90; anxiety after, 60–61; attention deficits after, 120; behavioral and environmental interventions for, 94; bleeding in brain due to, 25; cognitive behavioral therapy and, 63; cognitive deficits after, 117; delirium due to, 60; depression after, 41; executive dysfunction after, 133; headaches after, 150, 151; memory loss after, 126, 130; pseudobulbar affect after, 44; psychosis after, 83, 85; recovery after, 30, 34–35; seizures after, 81, 83, 85, 92, 155, 158, 160, 161; skull fracture and, 23; sleep problems after, 106; vision problems after, 163, 166, 167
severity of TBI, 1–2; impact on recovery, 30, 35; psychosis and, 83; seizures and, 158, 161; vision problems and, 166
sexual behavior, 17, 100
shame, feelings of, 173, 176, 178
shift work, 70–71, 108, 112
silent epidemic, 2, 3
Sinemet (carbidopa-levodopa), 77
singing, 143
skull fractures, 23–24
sleep aids, 109–10, 114
sleep apnea, 109, 110, 111, 112, 113, 115, 183
sleep disturbances, 29, 79, 106–16, 171; anxiety and, 57; causes of, 109–10; depression and, 40, 42, 55; diagnosis of, 112; mania and, 67, 70; treatment of, 113–14; types of, 110–12

sleep hygiene, 30, 55, 70, 114, 115–16, 154
sleep stages, 108–9
sleepwalking, 113
Snoezelen multisensory environmental therapy, 76
snoring, 106, 111
social functioning, 3, 101, 135, 137, 144
social media, 123
social support, 33–34
social withdrawal, 55, 83
soma of neuron, 10–11, 183
speech and language therapy, 39, 72, 122, 137, 144, 145
spinal cord, 10, 16
spinal roots, 10
sports injuries, 1, 2, 81, 99, 106, 129, 149
steroids, 106, 111, 168
stimulants, 76, 96, 115, 123, 130–31, 137, 145
"Stop, Think, and Act" rule, 104
stress hormones, 46, 49
stress reduction/management, 51, 69–70, 71, 152, 154
stroke, 46, 73, 167
subgenual cingulate, 44–45, 47
subthalamic nucleus, 18
suicidality, 41, 42–43, 47, 53, 56, 75
sumatriptan (Imitrex), 149, 152
support groups, 98, 175
supportive therapy, 51, 69
suprachiasmatic nucleus, 109
sympathetic nervous system, 10
symptoms. See specific symptoms
synapses, 10–11, 15, 183

talk therapy. See psychotherapy
TBI. See mild TBI; moderate to severe TBI; severe TBI; traumatic brain injury
Tegretol (carbamazepine), 49, 69, 96, 104, 161
telegraphic speech, 141
temporal lobes, 16, 18, 20; aggression and, 92–93; bleeding in, 24, 25, 39; contusions of, 23, 125; impulsivity

and, 100; language and, 142–43; mania and, 68; memory and, 19, 128; psychosis and, 84, 85; seizures in, 157, 158; vision and, 19, 20, 166
terminology, 7, 179–83
thalamus, 15, 17, 18, 59, 73, 108, 109, 121, 165, 166
thyroid stimulating hormone, 18
timetable/schedule of activities, 53, 55, 76, 102, 115, 122, 129, 136, 138, 172
Topamax (topiramate), 153, 160
tranquilizers, 32
transcranial magnetic stimulation (TMS), 50, 177
transient direct current stimulation, 50, 177
traumatic brain injury (TBI): definition of, 1, 183; influences on recovery from, 29–36; long-term effects of, 2; severity of, 1–2; types (mechanisms) of, 21–22; types of brain damage from, 22–28. See also mild TBI; moderate to severe TBI; severe TBI
The Traumatic Brain Injury Model Systems (TBIMS) program, 186
trazodone, 114
Tylenol (acetaminophen), 29, 152
types of TBI, 21–22

UAB-TBIMS Home Stimulation Program, 186
unilateral spatial neglect, 167

Valium (diazepam), 32, 62, 114
valproic acid (Depakote), 49, 67, 69, 96, 104, 153, 161
vegetative state, 35
venlafaxine (Effexor), 48, 62, 77
Veterans Health Information Clearing House, 188
Vicodin (hydrocodone/acetaminophen), 32, 92
vigilance, 61, 82, 120, 121, 183
visual problems, 28, 163–69; brain circuitry of, 164–67; tips for coping with, 168–69; treatment of, 167–68

visual processing, 16, 19, 20, 164–66
vocational rehabilitation, 122
vomiting, 28, 149, 150, 151, 154

weakness, 28
Wellbutrin (bupropion), 48, 77
Wernicke's area, 143
whiplash injury, 29
white matter of brain, 15, 26, 84–85, 183

Xanax (alprazolam), 32, 91, 114

yoga, 34, 63, 64, 103, 115, 152, 154

Zoloft (sertraline), 4, 47, 62, 96, 104
zolpidem (Ambien), 114
Zomig (zolmitriptan), 152
Zyprexa (olanzapine), 69, 85